D0935291

Bellevue Is a State of Mind

Anne Barry

BELLEVUE
IS A STATE
OF MIND

Harcourt Brace Jovanovich, Inc.

New York

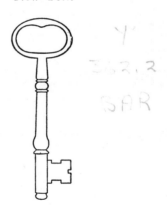

14858

Copyright © 1971 Anne Barry

All rights reserved.
No part of this publication may be reproduced
or transmitted in any form or by any means,
electronic or mechanical, including photocopy, recording,
or any information storage and retrieval system,
without permission in writing from the publisher.
First edition
ISBN 0-15-111750-0
Library of Congress Catalog Card Number: 72-153680
Printed in the United States of America

A B C D E

For Norman, with affection

Acknowledgments

This book describes a week spent on Ward N 7 in the winter of 1969. Its inhabitants have long since left for home, or for other hospitals, and some of them have been re-admitted to Bellevue. Some of the nurses and aides have been assigned to other wards or have taken jobs elsewhere. After my release, Bellevue became a teaching hospital associated with New York University; the organization of the psychiatric wards is different, there is a larger staff, there is a new emphasis on milieu therapy. When I was admitted, N 7 was still known as the violent ward, a concept now banished from Bellevue. In fact, within weeks of my departure, N 7 as I knew it ceased to exist.

I began this piece of research in seriousness, without much concern for topicality. N 7 could be any overcrowded, conventional, good psychiatric ward in any large American city. The problems of the patients often remain the same, no matter how rigid or innovative the particular hospital administration may be. The N 7 I knew was distinguished from other wards by being a little better than most; in many ways, the relationships between individuals, and between the patients and the institution, are universal.

I wish to thank The Very Reverend Michael Allen, Sandra Charlebois, Robert Davidson, Helen Brann, and Bruce Ennis for their particular and much needed help. Tony Mirkin, whom I met after my release, was generous with his time and interest. I was impressed with the tolerance and flexibility of Joseph Terenzio, then Commissioner of Hospitals, and of Dr. Alexander Thomas, Head of the Psychiatric Division at Bellevue, who accepted the news of my writing project, and the practical research that I had done, with equanimity. I thank the doctors on the ward who treated me when I was a patient, and then answered my questions in the months of writing this book. I have changed the names of aides, nurses, doctors, and patients at Bellevue to protect their privacy; for that reason alone I do not list them here, each one, in gratitude for their friendship and their help when I needed it. If any should read this book, I hope they will find in it clear evidence of my appreciation.

Bellevue Is a State of Mind

One

I was taken down a corridor, into a waiting room garish with bright lights. On wooden benches sat three drunks; one old lady with spiky hair muttering about her brother in Albany; a policeman, half asleep; a Puerto Rican man and woman restraining a girl in a filmy blue nightgown. The girl's hair was done up in a long braid hanging down below her waist. She was pulling the braid over her head and stuffing it in her mouth. This is where the police bring you in their ambulance, if you are picked up on the streets of Manhattan screaming stories at the crowd that gathers to watch you; this is where they bring you when they think you are insane. It was three o'clock on a cold February morning, at Bellevue Hospital. Only another half hour, maybe an hour, and I would be admitted to the psycho ward. I was very tired, for I had been trying to get in since 10:15 that evening.

Months before, I had planned to explore life at Bellevue, one of the oldest hospitals in the country, sprawling between the East River and First Avenue in the Kips Bay section of the city. The building that houses the psychiatric patients is a U-shaped brick fortress at Thirtieth Street; when you walk by, you see men at the second-floor windows, their hands gripping prison bars. I had thought about getting a job as an aide or as a volunteer, but when I thought about my motives, it was plain that I was interested less in the staff's point of view than the patients'. At the moment one lets go all restraints, abandons reason and all the ordinary rules, who is there to help, and what help could there be? Without rules, is there chaos, or perhaps a new odd set of rules that gets one through the straits of insanity, and sees to it one emerges alive? I wondered, too, what would be left to a person deprived of his position in the world, removed from family and friends, stripped of reputation, even of his clothes, a lock placed on the door. When his every word is disregarded, when he is not trusted, can he still feel that he is a free spirit? Can he find his own dignity, can he find allies? Will he love his wardens? Will he love his fellows, trapped with him out of reason, and out of mind? I decided to become a special sort of observer, an observer disguised as a patient.

For weeks I planned. I talked to doctors and lawyers, but for all of them it was impractical to back me openly in this project. Some offered help behind the scenes, but no doctor could sign me in, or (more important to me) sign me out. I would go ahead with it on my own. I did not know what danger, if any, lay ahead, so to spare my family, I kept the project secret. As a precaution, I told Michael Allen, then rector of St. Mark's in the Bowery, and my friend as well as my minister. I felt safer for his knowing what I was planning to do, and because he was a man of imagination, he gave me no arguments against it.

I knew I would need some liaison with the outside world, so I chose one other person that I trusted, a woman settled in the world, who would impress the hospital staff as both kind and competent, and asked her to pose as my only friend. Because I wanted to explore a typical route into Bellevue, and because I thought I might convince the law more easily than a psychiatrist that I was psychotic, I braced my friend Helen for a telephone call late one night from the police. I had heard enough stories of tough cops to scare me, but if this was to be an honest experiment, no compromises would do. Now I would find out for myself how and on just what provocation the police took a person to Bellevue. Would they be hasty, abusive, or kind?

At 7:00 P.M. on Friday, February 7, I took a bath, set my hair, and made myself ready like a sacrifice. In my pocketbook I put a few belongings, carefully chosen. I tucked in a Dostoevsky novel—*The Idiot*. (I wished with gallows humor that I had a paperback edition of *The Possessed*.) I had an old expired booklet from a time I had collected unemployment compensation, and that went into the pocketbook, too. It would be easiest to turn my "psychosis" on problems with finding work and holding a job. If I spun a tale of disordered personal relationships, I might inadvertently trip myself up, or reveal myself as merely neurotic.

Dexedrine, one of the commonest ups in a druggist's box of trips, used to be easy to come by; I knew a doctor once who gave me a prescription, endlessly refillable, to see me through college exams. Now, years later, I remembered that the bottle (unused since hallucinations caught me out in an all-night cafeteria in Harvard Square) was packed away in a drawer. Shortly before 10:15 I swallowed a ten-milligram spansule, to counteract the effects of any tranquilizers I might be given at Bellevue, and one five-milligram tablet, to see me through the next hours, and left my apartment with no idea when I would return.

I had to find a foot patrolman near enough to Bellevue to insure that I would be admitted there, yet at the same time far enough from my own neighborhood to avoid the police I saw every day on their beat, although it was unlikely that they would recognize me. The face that attracts a crowd is anonymous; who can describe the bank robber or the mugger? But I was stricken with a sort of modesty, and headed up First Avenue. I walked up to Twenty-third Street, then down Second Avenue as far as Tenth Street. Up Third Avenue, across Fourteenth Street. There was not a policeman in sight. I walked for an hour, then another half hour, hunching my shoulders and muttering, shooting hostile looks at passers-by. Now I considered that I knew nothing about acting (I who had forgotten my lines in every school play), and tried to remember everything I had ever read about Stanislavski, to get inside this new insane character. "Get away from me," I snarled, jumping as if someone had leaped at me from an alley. "Stop following me." Thus I progressed eastward, now scuttling sideways like a crab, now waving my arms. Doing well, I thought, until a voice asked, "Could you tell me the way to the Lexington Avenue subway?" I stammered directions. "Thank you very much," the woman said. I was underplaying it.

In a White Tower I had a cup of coffee to rev up the Dexedrine and reconsider tactics. It was impossible to find a policeman. I had come upon a patrol car stopped for a light, had run up and said, "There is a man who's following me," or tried to. The first three words came out stiff, as if I was reading them, and I fled. The car drove on. I felt angry and absolutely determined, and at the same time was embarrassed. Although I was grateful that passers-by didn't stare at me, I wondered why they didn't. I felt as conspicuous as Hyde.

I walked down to the Village, fighting my way through crowds on Bleecker Street. Surely here would be a policeman. "Stop following me!" I said as loudly as I could, twitching my arms and bumping into people. There was a cop on the corner. I began to talk loudly to myself; he laughed, and turned his back. I turned north again. It would have to be Washington Square Park.

The park was lonely. A couple locked together on a bench, two homosexuals holding hands by the empty fountain, and a policeman strolling around the periphery of the park, swinging his nightstick. "It's not my fault," I began conversationally, "and you spread lies." The policeman kept on walking. "Get away! Don't blame me for things I didn't do!" The policeman looked around once, then kept on moving. I ran up to him and pulled on his sleeve.

"Sir," I said, looking around in all directions, "there's someone following me. I can't stand it any more."

"Why don't you go home?" he said kindly. He was young, tall, and plump, with several chins, over which he peered at me with concern.

"I can't go home," I said in a hushed, conspiratorial tone. "He's there, too! He knows where I live, and if he gets into my house, I don't know what will happen!"

"What have you been taking?" the policeman asked. "Are you on LSD?"

"Of course not!" I was genuinely shocked. All my efforts mistaken for a bad trip!

"Do you want me to take you to a hospital?" the cop went on. "Do you want to talk to a doctor?" This was a bad turn. If I said yes, I might in effect be committing myself, which I did not want to do. I had thought the police might be easier to convince than hospital psychiatrists, but now I wasn't sure. The policeman did not believe me. He was baiting me. "Shall I take you to see a doctor?" he asked again. I moaned, fixed my eye over his shoulder, took on an expression of horror.

"He's there!" I whispered, and galloped away at full tilt.

Around the edge of the park, apartment windows were still lit—it was by now well after midnight—and looked warm and inviting. I remembered some friends who lived on Washington Square North, picked out their window, saw their lights on, wondered if they would pull aside the curtains and look out. Would they recognize me? Could they hear me? "The hell with it," I thought. It was getting cold, and I was tired. My arms and legs were sagging, and my body seemed held up by my heart, grown big as a grapefruit, hammering the Dexedrine through the arteries. I took a deep breath and began to scream until my voice cracked. It sounded like somebody else's voice. Some bystanders gathered. "Quit staring at me!" I yelled. "You're with him, I know you are!" They stopped to talk to the policeman. Scraps of conversation drifted across the quiet

7

park. "She's been yelling like that for an hour. Stay out of it, if you're smart." Enraged, I snarled like an animal, and bellowed again, "Stop following me!"

The policeman laughed. "It sounds like she's *looking* for somebody to follow her," he said. "Maybe she wants *me* to follow her."

I was getting hoarse. The people in the park had no faces for me; by now I had no shame, I felt I was almost invisible. It seemed that no matter what I did, no one would note it. I was completely isolated.

I was lonely and uncomfortable. I moved on to Eighth Street and University Place, a busy corner even late at night. People came out of a bar on the corner to see what was going on. Even while I was yelling, jumping around in half circles, swearing at passers-by, I was wondering how I could possibly be behaving in this way. Making a scene in public! Contorting the face, being ugly! Being abusive! For one wild moment I realized I had broken through, renounced generations of orderly lessons in civilized behavior. It was terrifying to cut loose, like a ship swinging adrift into open sea, but there was something close to exhilaration, too, for I felt my isolation from the staring crowd the way a captain might feel the swell of the ocean through the hull of his ship with its engines gone dead. The unspeakable had happened, other and mysterious forces had control, and now, paradoxically, I was totally free. I cried out, "I am not responsible! Let me be!" But the moment passed, that little glimpse of insanity, and I was wrapped up in loneliness as stifling as a blanket. I understood the feelings of a person who is very upset: the faces blur, one is anonymous, one has no name. One cannot communicate, one is surrounded by a wall. Nothing matters. If one shouts, no one hears. As I bellowed more curses on my demons, the crowd circled me without a word. They did not reach out. They stared with blank faces, their eyes as expressionless as holes punched in cardboard. I could not tell if they were angry, or concerned, or whether they thought of me as a diversion.

Then two or three faces came into focus. Someone did reach out. A boy of about eighteen said, "Hell, man, we've got to do something with her." Another said, "She's the same one that was in the park two hours ago." Five or six boys, friends looking for adventure in the Village, were gathered around me.

"Hey, stop yelling. You'll get into trouble. Don't yell, we'll get some help." An arm went around me, I was pressed clumsily against the boy's coat. "Don't be afraid," he said. "What's your name? We won't hurt you. You can talk to us. We won't let anybody get you. We'll keep him away."

"Cut it out, Marty, she's just a kook," said one of the other boys.

"My name is Anne," I whispered. The boy's coat was half open and he was wearing a grey Shetland sweater. He held me tighter and his chest felt as hard and flat as my younger brother's, and for a few moments I felt absolutely safe.

"Shut up," he said over my head. "We've got to do something with her."

Another boy said, "We can't find a cop. If we do, they'll slam us up against the wall for giving her stuff."

Marty asked me in a whisper if I had taken any drugs, had I been at a party? Did someone give me a pill to take? Or any cigarettes? No, no, no, I whispered back.

"She says she's not on drugs," he told his friends with a little uncertainty in his voice. "She's sick."

"Screw it. You can be a sucker if you want, but I'm splitting," a boy said. He left with all but Marty and one other boy, a red-headed extrovert with freckles. His name was Tom. Together they debated where to find a policeman. "There's bound to be one on St. Mark's Place," they decided. They marched me down Eighth Street, past Cooper Union, right through my neighborhood. Along the way I told Marty more of my story. The man kept following me, I said, but I had a secret plan to evade him. I looked wise and sly. I implied that the secret plan had something to do with razor blades or sleeping pills.

A right onto Second Avenue, and we came upon a policeman,

one I had spent a few minutes talking to only the night before.

"I don't think I like that policeman," I said as we approached him.

"Look, I'm with you." I buried my face in his sweater. "She's very paranoid, Officer. She was screaming about somebody following her for the last two hours. She told me she's been feeling like somebody's trying to get her for a couple of weeks."

"Don't get mixed up with it. Leave her alone. She could get you in a lot of trouble. What do you want to look for trouble for?"

"You've got to help her," Marty said.

Why were the police so reluctant to pick me up? I could imagine that they were only trying to be kind—who knows what hippie drug orgy they might stumble upon if they were to take me home, or what drugs they feared to find in my pocketbook. Perhaps screaming girls were now so common in New York that the jails and hospitals were filled up with them, leaving the law to gather in only the worst cases. It might be that the hospitals, overcrowded and understaffed, discouraged on-the-street lay diagnoses. I could see I put this policeman in a nice spot; one eye on my desperate face, he was wishing for something straightforward and clear, a burglar caught in the act, or a teen-ager joy-riding in a stolen car. Crazy people were out of his line. The policeman said, "What the hell, I can't do anything, but if you want, take her down to the Ninth Precinct, on Fifth Street."

That dingy building was humming with activity. At the big desk a rookie cop took calls. Behind a railing a sergeant said into the phone, "Are you going to make that assault with a deadly weapon, Artie? The guy says he doesn't want to press charges. What do you say?" A man in a Chesterfield coat waited his turn to report a stolen car. I was put on a wooden chair. The sergeant was stocky, grey-haired, and overworked. He asked the boys what drugs I was on. I was relieved the boys were with me, for I couldn't have acted out paranoia for the police. I was tearful and anxious and miserable. The boys explained about my screaming, my suicidal tendencies. The sergeant's eyes shot up. He gently took my pocketbook while I clung to Marty. They found the unemployment booklet, the driver's license. The rookie came over to see what was happening. "This license is no good. This girl is about fourteen, and the license says she's twenty-eight."

"I think it's hers," Marty said. They scrutinized my face.

"I guess it's okay. That's her." We went over once again that I lived alone, had neither relatives nor a job. Whenever I hesitated, Marty and Tom filled in details. I felt more withdrawn and frightened than I thought a sane person should; I didn't know whether or not I was putting on an act.

"Hey, look at this," the rookie said, unfolding a paper from my pocketbook. It was a letter I had written on lined notebook paper.

Dear Mayor Lindsay,

I am writing you because you are the only one who can help me with my problem. Someone is following me and I am afraid. People have spread stories about me that are not true. They say I was fired from my job but it wasn't my fault. Why don't you put more policemen on my block, to protect me. They call me on the telephone and say they are going to torture me.

P.S. I would like to see you in person because something has happened and only you will understand my problem.

"She must have been going to mail this," said the rookie.

"I don't know what to do with her," confessed the sergeant. "You don't want us to psycho her, do you? Christ, that's horrible, the psycho ward."

Marty said, "But what's wrong with this city, that it can't help someone who's sick and in trouble? Isn't there anybody who can help?" The question hung there, in a little pocket of silence—it was just chance that at that moment the telephone was still, the rookie was writing on a pad, the man in the Chesterfield was no longer drumming his fingers on the wooden railing; the words shifted the mood. They cut through the cigarette haze and the dust motes under the yellow light, and I

11

was not the only one thinking of questions larger than the cost of the stolen automobile, or the facts the rookie was putting into his report. The sergeant sighed. His shoulders sagged. He said, "Let me try one more time. Miss, don't you have anyone who could look after you tonight?"

Haltingly I mentioned Helen's name, and gave her telephone number. The sergeant scanned the letter to Mayor Lindsay again, shook his head, and turned to his desk to make the call.

"Miss Helen Miner? This is Sergeant Dagin, Ninth Precinct. We have a girl here. . . ." I couldn't hear the whole conversation because Marty was soothing me, telling me that the policemen were keeping the man who was following me out in the street. I caught a fragment, ". . . come down here, Miss Miner, and take her home."

"No," I cried out. "Keep her away from here. I don't want her down here. He'll follow her if she comes down here." I yelled hysterically and Marty looked scared. The police reassured me that Helen wouldn't be down tonight. I would see her the next day. "I want my letter back," I said in a tiny voice. "That is my property." They humored me, and I put it inside the unemployment booklet for safekeeping. The sergeant made another call. "No, no, she's not violent. Not now, anyway. But step on it, will you."

The lights in the station seemed a harsher yellow, the shadows hid creatures with eyes and thinking minds. My every muscle ached. The delusions had a life of their own; they shared my body with the mind of the objective observer. Acting was unnecessary. The police, even Marty and Tom, were nervous talking to me. They did not know precisely what tone to take. When I looked into their eyes I saw images of how they expected a psychotic to act; although I was sitting perfectly still, and had been for the twenty minutes since the telephone call to Helen, they saw me as close to violent. I told myself, "Nothing you do or say is going to be believed."

The ambulance arrived. Tom and Marty helped me into the back and sat with me. "Where are we going?" I asked.

The policemen exchanged looks. "To a place where you will

get some help," they said. "To a hospital." When I moved to look out the back window, the policemen jumped as if they were ready to hold me down. The city was a dark blur outside, punctuated by street lights. I couldn't see where we were going. "What hospital?" I was afraid perhaps I had been wrong, perhaps they could and would take me to Roosevelt or Metropolitan. My own helplessness was beginning to dawn on me. The policeman reluctantly said, "Bellevue."

We swung into what looked like a large alley, to a back door. I was helped out, and into a grim, shabby building. The boys stayed with me in the waiting room. They had by now been with me for hours, they were tired, and when they didn't notice my looking at them, they let their shoulders slump and their faces went soft and vulnerable. The three of us sat on bright-blue plastic chairs. The green rug was burned with so many stamped-out cigarette butts it looked as if it had a spotted pattern. The girl in the nightgown started to babble in Spanish and her relatives couldn't calm her. Remembering the paperback in my pocketbook, Marty asked me if I enjoyed Russian literature.

The boys went out into the corridor, by the main desk, to talk to a doctor. They were all looking at me and speaking with great animation. Marty came back and said, "We have to go now, but you're going to be all right. Don't worry. Your friend Helen will be here tomorrow to see you. Don't be afraid of anything."

It was now after 3:00 A.M. I was feeling lightheaded. "I like you," I said. Again the exhilaration of this license: I could say exactly what I felt like saying. "You're such a nice person. You're very kind, and you helped me, and I like you very much." Marty smiled and looked abashed. I threw my arms around him and hugged him as hard as I could. He, too, must have known that the usual rules were turned upside down, for instead of pulling away, he hugged me back, and then the boys left without saying goodbye.

I waited quietly for the nurse. The Puerto Rican girl was flinging her arms about and crying out. The nurse came up quickly, then another nurse, with a hypodermic. "Come now, be a good girl, calm down now," she said, as she expertly pushed the nightgown up. The man and woman helped hold the girl while she got the shot. She fell on the floor, was helped onto the bench, and a few moments later was led away. The Puerto Rican woman held the man's hand and started to cry.

My body moved closer to sleep, but the Dexedrine, on some schedule of its own, speeded my pulse with a lurch. In the corridor outside, four policemen sprawled on benches and watched me watching them. "Did you see those guys?" one of the policemen said to his friend. "One of them said, 'She's very paranoid,' and the other one said, 'She's psychotic, with suicidal tendencies.' I guess they thought they were fucking psychiatrists."

"She come from around here?"

"St. Mark's Place, or that's what they said."

"Ha. Is that where she lives or is that where she flops?"

"I don't know, they said they found her in the street."

"What do you bet those fuckers gave her pills? Banged her a few times, she took a bad trip, and then they dump her. Those cocksuckers looked scared shitless."

"Well, who gives a fuck. Joe, you get the coffee this time. Get me a container of light and a Danish."

A nurse came into the waiting room with a pill in a paper cup. "You aren't going to make me give you an injection, are you?" she said. I swallowed the pill, she grasped my arm firmly above the elbow and led me past the policemen and down the long corridor to a small office. I hesitated in the doorway like an animal being cajoled into a cage.

"Come in, come in," said the doctor. It had been a long night for him. Here was the fourth new admission in an hour, and it was almost 4:00 A.M. He was young, and impatient. He wore his doctor's coat with an air of importance. He had a small tidy mustache. "Sit down," he said.

I sat on the edge of a chair at the corner of his desk. He opened a file folder in front of him. After routine questions

14

about my name and age and address, he leaned forward in an attitude of compassion. "Just why are you here, Miss Barry?"

"The police brought me. Some boys brought me, and then the police. I was afraid, and I got upset."

"Just why were you upset?"

Silence. He glanced into the folder.

"Did you think someone was, uh, following you, Miss Barry?"

"Yes," I whispered. "I couldn't see his face. He wears a floppy hat with a big brim—" I gestured vaguely in the air to show the width of the brim.

"Has he been following you long?"

"A couple of weeks. He calls me on the telephone. I think he knows where I live."

"Come, come, Miss Barry. You must speak a little louder. I can't hear you. Have you taken any drugs tonight, Miss Barry?"

"No, never anything like that."

"Tell me about your family, Miss Barry. Do you have any relatives in the city?"

"No, there's only Helen. Helen is my friend."

"Have you ever been approached by a woman, Miss Barry?" I had no idea what he was talking about. "For sexual purposes?" he added. "Tell me about Helen," as if the two subjects were the same.

I started to improvise. I looked him in the eye and spun lies, wondering if my red cheeks or guilty expression gave him a clue that I wasn't telling the truth. "She knew my family when I was a little girl. I met her out in Colorado. She helped me get a job one time. When I first came to New York. She sort of keeps an eye on me, now that my parents are dead."

"And what does she ask in return?"

"What?"

"I said, 'What does she ask in return?'" He peered narrowly at me, his pen poised above my chart to write down my reaction. The textbook I had studied hadn't told me lesbianism was an adjunct of the symptoms I had chosen. In none of those case studies had the patient been homosexual. I had only

15

seconds to decide whether to discourage this impression, or strengthen it; I hadn't had any experience in that line, but perhaps to fake it would insure that I was speedily admitted. I was beginning to wonder if I seemed upset enough. I had been sounding too calm and logical to be truly psychotic. But pretending to be a lesbian would require concentration; I was so tired, my thoughts were in fragments. Worse, I suddenly doubted my heterosexuality. I hadn't in the past, but perhaps, like a witch, he would pull from me some response that led to mysteries sleeping for years, waiting for just this man and just this course of dialogue. I was ready to believe anything.

"I don't know what you mean."

"Well, let it go," the doctor said. After a moment he began to write in the folder. "Try to co-operate, Miss Barry. We're only trying to help you." He sat back, bored. Perhaps I had made a mistake; he was losing interest and would soon decide I didn't require admission at all.

"And how do you feel, Miss Barry?" He spoke pleasantly, as if picking up a conversation with a casual friend at a cocktail party.

"I'm very frightened."

"Still frightened, eh?" He was amused. He took out a stethoscope and placed it under my shirt. He listened, listened again. Moved it about and listened some more. The Dexedrine I had taken was pounding like a fist. His expression changed. He wrote rapidly for some minutes. He listened again with the stethoscope. "You certainly are frightened," he said in a different voice. "We think that you should stay here so that we can help you, Miss Barry. We want to see that the man doesn't try to follow you any more. We'll make sure he goes away." Although he was making an effort to sound kind and sympathetic, he let the effort show as if he wanted me to thank him for it. Or he thought I was too dull-witted to notice.

The nurse reappeared to lead me off to a small room crowded with cupboards and closets. The aide was leaning through the door to the next room to talk to another hospital worker. Their

16

conversation interrupted her business with me, and a simple transaction was thus protracted into a rite.

The aide plucked items from my pocketbook and listed them on a form. One unemployment book. Four postage stamps. One driver's license. Two pencils. These were put in a pile. I couldn't follow the conversation with the man in the next room; I concentrated hard on each word, but they wouldn't form sentences in my mind. I heard something about Sophia Loren and her baby. My heart kept pounding. Maybe a heart could break open if it beat hard enough. I started to count the thumps I heard in my eardrums. Now the two were talking about a book the aide wanted to read. He said no, he didn't want to read no book she says he's got to read. She asked him what kind of books he liked to read, and he said books like *True Detective*. I was working hard not to fall over in the chair. The man called the aide Eloise. Eloise said he was too dumb to read anything except girlie books. It was twenty minutes past four. Closing my eyes made me more dizzy. Thud, thud, thud, thud. My heart filled up my chest, it choked me, there was nothing left of my body but my heart.

My mind was disappearing, too. Every time the woman flicked her fingers over my money, my papers, even my pencils, she dismembered my mind. A pile for the property we lock up *for* you. A pile for the property we lock up *with* you. One you can't have, one you can. How could she be touching my property, and paying so little attention to it, or to me? My property! It was all I had. She picked up my paperback book.

"I'm reading a book, too," I said, concentrating on making sense.

"What?" she said, as if I was not making sense.

"You told that man you were reading a book. I was wondering what the name of it is."

"Oh, *The Pearl*." She was for the first time aware that I had heard a conversation taking place three feet away from me.

"I'm reading that book you're holding," I said, bound to civility. This was the first time I was desperately polite to a

17

staff member who considered me a nuisance, but later I saw that most of the other patients reacted just the same way. The courteous have dignity, and sometimes a patient has only this to fall back on.

The aide said, "Well, I guess you can keep the book. Take it up to the ward with you. You can't have this comb. It's got this long pointed handle on it. You can't have the pencils." She started on the second pile. "You can have your change purse, and I'll put one of your dollars in it, in case you want to buy cigarettes. When you need more money, you just ask for it, and they'll take it from the other three dollars." I remembered the letter to Mayor Lindsay I had tucked into the unemployment booklet, and asked for it. "It's my property," I said. She gave me the paper without reading it, and I put it inside the pages of the paperback. I found myself inordinately grateful to her for allowing me any property at all.

She asked me if I had ever been hospitalized. Did I have any identifying marks or scars? No to both questions. "Take off your clothes," she said, putting a screen across the open doorway where the male attendant was sitting. "You can keep your bra and panties." She took my blue jeans, my coat, my jersey one by one and put them on a hanger inside a large white bag. My shoes were tossed in, my empty pocketbook. She gave me a heavy cotton dress with a windowpane check of yellow and red; a green and white seersucker robe; and slippers like clown feet, with huge cardboard soles and floppy mesh uppers elasticized around the ankle. Each garment was stenciled BELLEVUE across the front in letters two inches high. The dress was very long and tied at the back. The waistline swung below my hips. Eloise put the possessions I was not allowed to have in a box. What a sense of loss! I felt unrelated to myself.

"Did I ask you if you have any identifying marks or scars?" Eloise asked.

"No scars."

"When it's late like this, you know, sometimes I forget what I'm doing. This is the damnedest shift."

If I should die right now, I thought, they would have to

18

check my teeth in the morgue to trace who I am. No identification at all! But Eloise reached out and put around my wrist a plastic bracelet with my name on a label. "Now you can't get lost." The bracelet was so designed that it could be removed only with scissors or a knife.

Eloise passed me on to a nurse who took me up in an elevator as large and gloomy as a freight elevator. We emerged on the seventh floor. The walls of the hallway had been freshly painted off-white, the doorways were new harsh colors—pink, purple, orange, and brown—the paint thick and shiny over the uneven, pockmarked layers of previous coats. We faced a locked door, painted purple. A key big as the keys to old New England houses let us in. To our right, another locked door, leading to the men's ward, O 7, and to the left, a locked door leading to the women's ward, N 7. Inside, dim lights in the ceiling showed a corridor that turned a right angle thirty feet from us, and in that area aides were sitting around a card table. They gathered around me, asked a question or two of the nurse, and put me in a bed in the hallway. For company I had three other patients in beds end to end; we were the new admissions kept in the corridor for observation during the night.

It was hard to go to sleep because the Dexedrine still spun through my bloodstream. Shrieks of laughter from the aides woke me whenever one of them told a joke. The steam heat hissed. The ward was overheated; I sweated as if on the edge of fever. I fell into an uneasy doze, but within an hour, it was morning.

Two

At 7:00 A.M. the ward was awakened by an aide bellowing, "Breakfast, ladies!" We were a motley collection of women, frowsy, pale, vacant-eyed. We were always called ladies, and picked up the term ourselves with no sense of irony. I was nervous here for unexpected reasons. I couldn't help wondering if some patient, or a sadistic aide, would attack me, or if a doctor might throw me into shock treatment by mistake, but I had worried over these bad chances so often in the last weeks, they had no hold on me and seemed abstractions. I had expected to be afraid, and prepared myself. It was almost an anticlimax now to run through the possibilities and find them all impossible, at least for the moment. These ghosts, my wardmates, stumbling along the hall on the way to the bathroom, hawking and spitting into the basins, crouching over the toilets in their doorless stalls, seemed far from violent. A real fear sprang from my newness here. The patients knew the ward routine, they knew their limits. I was surprised by a kind of envy of these women who did not question their dreary surroundings. I was all the more adrift here for being sane, and self-conscious about how I got here. The threat lay more in my own rationality than in my ward-mates' madness, for they belonged here, and I didn't.

"Get your ass out of bed, ladies!" the aide yelled, and I found my way to a chair outside the bathroom holding a tray of Lavoris in paper cups. I wanted to do everything right, just like a patient. The bathroom had eight washbowls, each with a mirror made of shiny unbreakable metal. Two of the bowls had hot and cold water, but all the rest had the spigots removed and capped. Beyond the bowls were the four toilets, all occupied. Lying on the floor pressing her back against the wall was a young girl, silent, eyes rolled back. Everyone ignored her, so I tried to ignore her, too.

I washed as best I could without toothbrush or towel and followed the other patients out to the corridor. My bed was gone. I had left my bathrobe on the end of the bed, and so it, too, was gone, with my change purse in the pocket, and my book. The last of my possessions, gone! Another terrific sense of loss. There was nothing left of me at all. The aides were busy rousing slow patients from the dormitory rooms and bundling them into the bathroom, accompanying their actions with blunt directives, not unkindly given. "Get your ass out of bed, Miss Jenks. How you going to get out of here if you don't shape up? Now Miss Hargins, look at that mess you made. You *pick* that cup up there. Don't you throw nothing on the floor. You there, yes, you. You taking too long washing up. You clean enough. How's the other ladies going to get washed, if you're sitting in that bowl like that?"

I moved down to the area that became an improvised day room—the space where the corridor made a right angle. There patients were sitting on orange plastic chairs, lined up, a row against each wall. I sat down, too, to wait with them for breakfast.

The ladies were at first faceless. There were thirty or thirty-five on the ward, although it was hard to make an estimate. Some were locked off in other rooms, or on the toilet, or sleeping; by the time I counted one area, those women had drifted away, replaced by others. They looked alike in their hospital gowns. They looked alike with their sad, expressionless faces. Gradually one or two ladies, livelier than the rest, began to stand out.

"All right, ladies, who plugged up the fountain?" a tall stringy woman called in a Midwestern twang. "Whoever plugged up the fountain, come help me dip the water out of it. Who put shit down the fountain to plug it up?" It sounded like a parody of an aide's tone of voice. The woman nagged us along like children. "All right, who's going to clean the bathroom? Somebody has to clean the bathroom. Somebody has to clean the toilets and somebody has to clean the sinks. Gerta, you can be an inspector today if you want." A German girl in her late twenties said, "Okay, Norma June, today I inspect if you want me to," then caught my eye and giggled. Norma June's voice was so harsh it was an offense. I was grateful for her, nonetheless, for she knew some rules here, or made them up, and how the others responded to her might give me some clue toward how to act myself. But most of the patients sat silent, not looking at her. I acted as if I were ignoring her, too. "Priscilla, you going to clean the toilets? I bet you're the one who plugged up this damn fountain. You should be ashamed of all this shit." She was talking to the girl I had seen lying on the bathroom floor. Priscilla didn't answer.

"You have a big mouth, woman," someone said.

"All right, I'll shut up then. I know I talk too much." But two minutes later she was roaming up and down the hall, and her voice carried the length of the ward. "How are you this morning, Mrs. Weldon, you're looking very pretty this morning, and how are you, Leola, don't your hair look nice the way it's done up today."

A lady shook her head. "That Norma June. She just has a big mouth, but I guess she can't help it."

"She's nice, though," the woman sitting next to her answered, after thinking about it. "She's got a good heart."

"Who's making all that noise? Who the fuck is yellin'?" Swaggering down the hall came a short girl with thick black hair cut in an Elvis Presley ducktail. Pale skin and big black eyes gave her a vulnerable look that she counteracted by swinging her shoulders like a man when she walked, and by talking tough out of the side of her mouth. "I'm a Sicilian," she called out. "I'm a Sicilian and I'm tough. I don't take nothin' from nobody." I wasn't about to get in her way. First the doctor last night, with his smug insinuations, and now Phoebe Dagostino. I had expected drug addicts and whores, but dykes were another matter. There was little relation between the textbook I had studied and real life on the ward. It was something to think about.

At 8:00 A.M. we were called into the dining room, a large room painted white over what close inspection showed to be tiles. It looked as if at one time this had been a shower room. Now it was filled with stainless-steel tables seating four or eight, and stainless-steel benches, and the orange-seated chairs. The food was served in blue plastic bowls. The only utensil was a large spoon, with a bowl an inch and a half across. This first morning the food looked repellent. The eggs were cold, the oatmeal cooked with water and transparent around the edges. I risked the coffee, which was cold, and the canned orange juice. I was sitting at a table with seven other ladies, most of them old, some of them slopping and spilling their food.

Periodically a cry went up—"Who wants my cereal? Does anybody want my eggs? There's a cup of coffee here if anyone wants it." Norma June started this trading of bowls and cups. She liked to make presents of anything in her possession. There were no second helpings, so this trading fulfilled a need. Many patients ate their breakfast with relish. The meal

23

was over in fifteen minutes. The little old lady with spiky hair whom I had seen in the waiting room was talking into the air about her brother the architect in Albany. There were plates of bread on the table, and pats of margarine, and envelopes of salt and sugar. The old lady took a dozen pieces of bread and made sandwiches with margarine, and concealed them under her nightgown. She walked out, looking lumpy, to sit in corners and nibble at the food behind her hand.

I set out to find my bed. The nurse's aides roamed the corridors, swinging beds around like stevedores. They called out, "Make your beds, ladies! Everybody get your linen and make up your beds!" The ladies crowded around the cart. I got there too late to find a pillowcase, but it didn't matter, because they were short of pillows, too.

"Where is my bed?" I asked an aide.

"I don't know, honey. How the hell should I know? Why don't you go look for it?"

I had inspected some fifteen beds when Norma June Jacobsen shouted, "Here's your bed, right in my room. That's real nice, you're right next to me. I like you, even if you don't talk much. Listen, everybody, this here is a nice girl. She don't talk much because she's scared, she's new here, but she'll get a lot better soon. Everybody be nice to her." And sure enough, there in a room containing just three beds was mine, with my robe at its feet, the change purse in the pocket, and underneath, untouched, my paperback book. My possessions in hand! I resolved never to be parted from them again. I felt stilted and shy with Norma June, as if she had in turn made me her property, but upon reflection, that was all right with me. I was unsure of myself, and she had seen it better than I, and had helped me.

"Showers, ladies! Get in line now, get moving, ladies!" A ragged line formed outside a room with one large shower stall built into the wall. We were herded in, in groups of four or six, and passed through the shower two at a time. As two washed, others were drying themselves or getting clean nightdresses. The air was so thick with steam we were damp before we stood under the showerhead, and the towels we dried ourselves with were clammy. Particularly obvious in the shower room was a peculiar, pervasive smell, redolent of sweat and psychosis, which most of us gave off and which could never be masked, although an aide passed around Ban roll-on for those who wished to try. No one commented on it; you live in dread and you breathe in the odors of dread. Psychosis has a smell of its own that you never forget.

There were smells here, and sights for the eye. Never before had I been surrounded by so many naked bodies. What shapes! What variety! I was jostled by pendulous breasts, buttocks turned crepy with age, skin that sagged, bellies that drooped. What differences of color! What symphonies of form! Body hair kinky or limp, in skimpy patches or swinging like beards, nipples black, brown, pink, and rose. Hips, breasts, stomachs, the curve of the spinal column—a dozen variations on the circle, the oval, the reverse curve. I watched my body in a scratched metal mirror for some moments before I recognized it as mine, it was so unfamiliar in this company. I felt no kinship with it—no identifying marks or scars. But I was pleased to see that it looked young and healthy and firm. It might have belonged to anyone.

In the shower room a slender pretty girl helped the aides hand out gowns and robes. She looked like the leader of a high-school gang outside, the trend setter, the girl who wore the shortest skirts and hid a transistor radio among her school books. Her skin was a smooth deep brown, and her expression was lively. Her eyes flashed with humor. Her self-confidence overwhelmed me and I felt shy with her, and as grateful for the robe she gave me as if she had been a member of the staff.

Still damp (by the time I had taken my shower, the towels were used up), we filed out into the corridor to sit. Mrs. Weldon, a middle-aged black woman with a face as lined and sad as a bloodhound's, sat near me, moaning over and over, "Lawd, lawd, oh me."

The staff nurses came on duty at 9:00 A.M. One of them,

Miss Sendell, young and blond, with a short skirt and granny glasses, asked me how I felt. She smiled at me. "Don't be frightened. The ward takes a little getting used to, but it's not really frightening."

She was right, of course. The patients moved quietly—it was partly the drugs, for most of us took Thorazine four times a day. We moved in slow motion. The depressed patients were particularly withdrawn, but even agitated patients seemed to try to subdue their reactions. There seemed to be a special ambience in the ward, a gentleness between the patients based on concern for one another's feelings.

It wasn't much after 10:00. The Dexedrine was losing to the Thorazine and lack of sleep the night before, and although my eyes were wide open, alert, my body felt halfway into sleep when I sat in a chair. I headed for the dormitory rooms to try to take a nap. I didn't hear the soft steps behind me because the cardboard slippers muffled the sound, and the girl stepped lightly. I was past the bend in the corridor where the nurses could see what was going on when a smooth arm slid around my neck from behind. I stopped walking. It must have been the gentle mood among the ladies on the ward that kept me from screaming; I was scarcely startled. I thought, "I mustn't make a sound. Everything will be all right if I don't scream." The arm pressed me tighter around the throat, then relaxed and turned me half around. It was Luisa, the Puerto Rican girl in the blue nightgown in the waiting room the night before. There was no violence in her eye; she was perfectly calm. In absolute silence she stroked my cheek, held me for what seemed like minutes. I surprised myself by patting her back awkwardly and saying, "There, there, you're a nice girl, don't be afraid," as touched and as clumsy as the two boys who had brought me into Bellevue. We clung to one another like two sisters. I couldn't remember the last time I had hugged a woman, yet here I was being comforted by a stranger. I wished I had Miss Sendell's confidence that there was after all nothing for us to be afraid of. Luisa murmured something in Spanish and moved on like a sleepwalker. Her almond eyes were staring ahead, but her attention was turned inward. Her long shining hair hung down her back in a braid like a rope.

I had lost all interest in sleep, so sat in the corridor to watch the ceaseless ebb and flow of shuffling ladies, up and down the hall, and the purposeful nurses hurrying about their duties. The ward was so small, there were few places to go. At one end of the corridor, a handful of rooms crowded with beds, then the bathroom, and the room where we took showers. My back was to the dining-room doors. To my right, the social workers' office. An office for nurses. The locked purple door. We seemed as busy as ants filmed in slow motion, moving from one side of our hill to the other, intent upon tasks. Because from either end of the corridor one could see only dirty beige walls broken by bright painted doors, one searched for variety. I began to think that other people must be enjoying friendships, conversations, sound advice in the dormitory when I prowled the corridor, in the dining room while I lingered outside the social workers' office—always just out of my reach. One imagined that obscured by the right angle of the corridor something of interest was happening. Doors offered promise. A corner might hide a secret. To be in motion, walking to and fro, implied a destination and therefore gave hope.

Moving about like this made me feel inconspicuous. Sometimes I sat still in a chair and practiced appearing withdrawn. I was terrified of being recognized. A doctor might at any moment pass through, narrow his eyes at me alone in the crowd of women, and say, "You, there. You shouldn't be here; you're perfectly well." Because I was acting out paranoia, I began to feel somewhat paranoid. Whenever the door opened and closed, when I heard the key turn in the lock, I felt: people are working against me, they are depriving me of my freedom.

I made plans to avoid telephones that might have unseen listeners in the hospital, to smuggle things in and out through visitors; when in fact I knew that the hospital staff was overworked, would not dream of taking the time to eavesdrop,

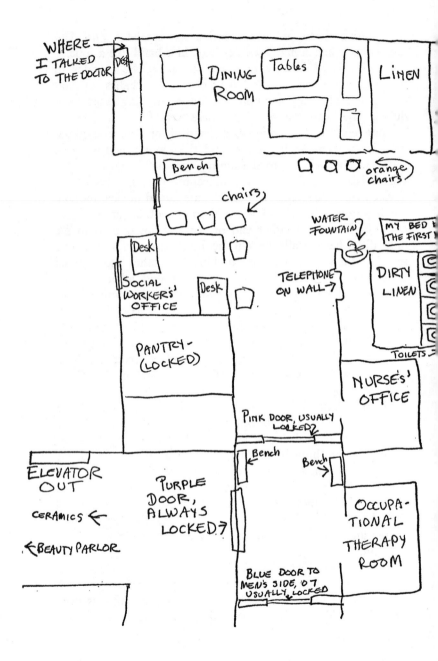

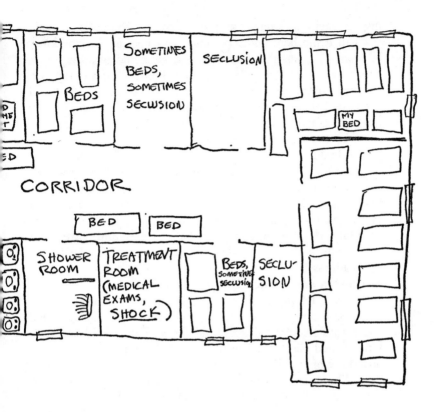

SOMETIMES BEDS, SOMETIMES SECLUSION

SECLUSION

BEDS

MY BED

CORRIDOR

BED   BED

SHOWER ROOM

TREATMENT ROOM (MEDICAL EXAMS, SHOCK)

BEDS, SOMETIMES SECLUSION

SECLUSION

WARD N 7
BELLEVUE

inspect packages brought by friends, or read the patients' mail.

I had come here under pretense, and because I alone knew how amazing was the deception, I alone could imagine others deceiving me on just so large a scale. I had unpinned my own moorings by coming here. No one looked more innocent and frightened than I, but if my presence here was trickery, others might be equally tricky. Surely the patients suspected me. That must be the reason they seemed to avoid me. I tried to surprise a huddle of women plotting against me. From the end of the corridor they looked to me like cabalists. But one was hallucinating, three were silent, one was asking no one in particular about her medication, and they were as unaware of me as they were of each other. They were not talking about me at all. Only Mrs. Foster, small and hard as a walnut, gave me a salute. She looked to be the only rational soul in the group; her madness took her like fits of an hour's or a day's duration. In between one wondered why she was here.

Before I let my anxiety frighten me away from the other patients, I remembered the larger dangers we shared. There was always that locked door, and the staff who held the keys. I mistrusted the staff, because they held me captive and deprived me of the slightest control over my actions. At the same time, like a half-remembered voice drifting across a span of years, I heard something calling me back to childhood again. I could not make out the words, just the tone, soothing and making no demands. I wanted to be taken care of. I would like an aide to stroll down the corridor with her arm around my shoulders, as I saw Miss Pinero walk with the young girl from the shower room. If the hospital administration was smart, it would plant such loving staff members to co-opt the patients and put down revolution. There were power alignments here, I was sure of it, and yet every combination I imagined left me with no allies at all. Any trust might be betrayed.

I shrank down in an orange chair. I hoped no one would notice me because I was not ready to respond to anyone. The more I tried to schematize this ward and my place in it, the more frightened I became. I returned to the reasons I came here. I wanted to be an observer, not a participant. I wanted to see what it felt like, but now that I was here, those very feelings were getting in my way; they were corrupting my judgment. I could not evaluate, because I had lost track of values. It had seemed reasonable to come here, see stimulus and response, attitude and theory, its practical application, the purposes and effects of drugs administered and how the patients responded to the efforts to help them. I had supposed that I would be set off from the patients only by my sanity, but here in fact the boundaries between us shifted like the line of battle in a guerrilla war. It didn't ring true to me, but to keep off hysteria I settled on this rigid pattern: here were well people and sick people. I was well, the staff was well, therefore they would let me function as a well person. They must know me for someone like them. When I comforted myself thus, I felt superior to the patients, and almost expected a staff member to hand me an aide's blue uniform and ask me to lend a hand.

These hours were a time of preparation. I would have to get through an interview with the doctor on Monday, face a young social worker and I didn't know how many others who were dedicated to helping me; I had to tell lies to them and I might surprise myself by telling the truth. Would they immediately release me? Would they suggest I go to a state hospital? I would catch myself working through fears not so very different from those of the real patients, and I would be brought up short by our similarity. Truly invisible, I sat with other invisible women, each on her own private journey, taking what she needed from inside herself, oblivious to what went on around her. A yoga could not have been immersed in a deeper meditation than I. Ideas, emotions, drifted in and out of my consciousness, overlapped, supplemented one another like the instruments in an orchestra. Like a leitmotif Luisa's blank eyes would be on me again, whether in fact or in memory I was not always sure, as if (if she could speak to me) she could answer a question I did not yet know how to ask.

From time to time some of the ladies would make tentative gestures to get to know me. A little old lady with frizzy hair said, "Good morning! Your head is on upside down!" and laughed. The German girl, Gerta, showed me what she had been making in occupational therapy. "It's a beach tote. I think it's very useful." It was a large cotton bag that held not her bathing cap but her few belongings here in the hospital. Recalling how close I had come to losing mine, I planned to investigate the occupational therapy room as soon as such an interest would be appropriate to my case. Gerta said, "I like it here very much. The nurses are so nice, and the food is very good." She sounded as if she were evaluating the service at the Plaza, and at first I thought she was joking. She told me that she had been a clerk for a company that made computers, but that now her job was gone. She had been here a month, and expected to leave soon. "I was terrible when I came in here, just terrible. You would not believe. I make a terrible noise, and shouting. I get better very quick, though."

There was something of the spinster about her; although she was younger than I she seemed years older. Her lips were too thin, her nostrils too pinched for charity. Life had not been generous to her, and she had been keeping accounts, she knew what was owed her. I could imagine the years in the tidy one-room apartment in good order, an orderly life, until one crazy night when she let the control loosen only a little (she didn't realize her mistake), and the whole thing blasted apart like fireworks. Sick, they said she was. Well, that was better than crazy, she shouldn't like to think of herself as crazy, because there was no alternative to crazy. But to be sick—one could then hope to be well; how much simpler. Gerta said, "The doctor thinks I'm doing very nicely. I'm going to leave soon, when I am well, but I'm feeling much better already. I like it here very much, but I will not be very sorry when I leave. But the staff is so nice. This is I think the best hospital." She said these things almost by rote, and I had no idea whether or not she was trying to convince herself by convincing me.

"It seems like a nice place," I said mildly. I looked at the dingy hall, the dirt in the corners, the gloom, and didn't think it was a nice place at all.

As if answering my thought, a woman in a dirty blue bathrobe passed me by with her eyes welling with tears. She was middle-aged, and if her eyes had not been puffy from crying, she would have been handsome. Her short thick hair was coal black except along the part. There, for the width of an inch, was a streak of white so striking that it looked intentional. One of the nurses had pointed her out earlier as Mrs. Zélie Briggs, a new patient like me, also hauled in after midnight. The white streak was vivid as a flag of distress; it must have been weeks since Mrs. Biggs had bothered to keep an appointment with a hairdresser. "Whatever you're grieving for, dear, I'm grieving with you," she said. "You don't know how terrible this experience has been. The best I can say is that it's going to come to an end. I know everything is going to be over soon." Her chin started to tremble.

A cheerful young black woman called after her, "Keep the faith, darlin', keep the faith. You got to pray to see light—I spoke to Jesus Christ about you, and that's his message. He says to tell you to keep the faith."

If only I had something to do, something to occupy my time! If I had been able to keep a pencil with me, perhaps I could have found a piece of paper somewhere and made some notes on my surroundings; I knew an ex-convict once who had written a novel in jail on hundreds of cigarette wrappers slipped to him by the other prisoners. I wanted to remember each person here—the drug addicts, the old women, the black girl six months pregnant, the alcoholics, the hypochrondriacs, and above all, the schizophrenics, who talked in their own private language. I asked Miss Sendell if one could write a letter here. "Come to the nurses' office and I'll give you a pencil, a piece of paper, and an envelope," she said. "When you're finished, give them all back to me, and I'll mail the letter for you."

Scant help there. For all I knew, they would watch me while

31

I wrote the letter, or at the least keep track of how long I kept the pencil. Paper would be another problem. I flipped through my copy of *The Idiot*, and couldn't concentrate on the print. But there, right in hand, was my paper! I could write on the margins, the flyleaves, the part titles, and no one would ever know. I tried to figure a way to steal a pencil from a nurse's pocket. It was hopeless.

I remembered that Helen would be coming to see me at visiting hours, and if I could somehow call her before she left home, she could bring me a pencil, and I could secrete it somewhere after she left. The pay telephone on the wall outside the nurses' office was for the patients' use, but it was out of order. "When will it be fixed?" I asked an aide. She laughed. "Honey, that phone is always broken. They get it to work, and two hours later it's broken again. You look close and I bet you see spider webs all over it, it's been so long since anybody called out on it." Again I had the desperate feeling of being locked in. At this point I didn't care if a nurse monitored calls, I'd settle for someone outside to do my calling for me, anything. But the aide added, "You can make one call after lunch and one call after dinner on the social workers' phone, and it won't cost you the dime. They allow that special privilege because of the phone being generally broken, but it's supposed to be just the poor folks that don't have any dimes that call for free. You line up between one and two o'clock."

I knew that by then Helen would be on her way to the hospital. "Is there any way I can make my call now? It's just a short one. I want my friend to bring me some things when she comes."

For twenty minutes I was passed from one aide to another, and on to the practical nurse, a clinician, the head nurse, and back to an aide with permission to use the telephone. It sat on one of the two desks in the office. I dialed 9 to get an outside line, so there was no way the call could be monitored through the supervisor's office, but I spoke in a strained, tense voice in case an aide was listening in the corridor outside. From time to time people would wander in and out of the office; there

32

was no closing the door for privacy. I sounded sick and halting. For her part, Helen asked me guarded questions that could be answered yes or no. We might have been acting in a World War II spy movie. I chose a moment carefully and quickly asked her to bring in a pencil, some fruit, and a toothbrush.

For lunch at noon we faced an anonymous hash and a salad of grated raw carrots and raisins. Like all meals here, it was over in fifteen or twenty minutes, leaving time like an abyss before the 2:00 visiting hour. I did not know how I would react to seeing a familiar face from my other world, whether I would start to giggle or find it impossible to keep up pretenses. Helen arrived looking out of place in a well-cut tweed coat and a Liberty scarf. I was so happy to see her, I almost cried. We went into the dining room, where all the patients were required to take their visitors, and found two seats slightly away from the others.

There was a great hubbub in the room as a dozen small dramas unfolded simultaneously—women laughed, scolded, wept at their husbands or parents. Each visitor was an event, and the patients' reactions were out of balance. The visitors made a colorful crowd. Here in the ward we had lost our social identities, but our visitors tended to reveal them. Seedy old men with frayed collars, clerk-typists on lunch hours, laborers in coveralls. The hippie boyfriend of an eighteen-year-old schizophrenic, in shoulder-length hair, dew band, and beads. Norma June's gaunt and kindly husband, with presents of the Life Savers and bubble gum she loves, and gives away.

Helen and I talked in low tones. I had to be careful of the expression on my face—I tended to look too animated. I must seem uncertain, almost shy. She handed me a paper bag with some toilet articles inside, and some fruit. We didn't know if packages were inspected, so Helen broke a stub off the pencil inside her pocketbook (it was loud as a rifle's crack—surely someone had heard, and would ask us about it! But no one noticed) and wrapped it in a dollar bill, and handed it to me with a great show. It just fit my change purse. When it was safely in my pocket Helen said she would talk to the social worker about my case as well as to the doctor, and then would slip me cues on how to behave after she found out how I was doing.

After Helen left I sank once again into gloom. Behind the locked door I felt artificial and amputated. All the tricks and games that got me through the days outside made no difference here—and part of the depression was realizing just what things propped me up outside. I enjoyed cleverness, wit, cerebration, and in the past had thought these were amusements. Now I saw that they took up time for me, I had given them a value out of proportion to their worth; and none of this had a thing to do with Norma June, or Gerta, or Luisa's loving embrace. In truth, my plotting with Helen now seemed a shabby trick, and I didn't know why. It had seemed such a good idea when I had first thought of it. That was the problem—it had been an idea to work out like a crossword puzzle, and I hadn't counted on my own feelings. My intellect had pinned me securely in the outside world, but these crazy people, cut adrift from reality, seemed more vivid to me here than I did to myself. I had thought that here I could analyze all the evidence as in a laboratory, but instead, becoming a part of the experiment, I had lost control. I couldn't remember precisely why I had come here.

One of the two doors was unlocked during the afternoon so that the men from O 7 could visit. Four or five men in blue pajamas and striped bathrobes watched television or played cards with Phoebe and Evelyn, the girl who had helped with the showers. The men made me uneasy. "Hi, baby," one said. "My name's Eddie. You want to play cards? You want to talk? Let's play checkers. I can teach you how to play poker. Maybe you'll give me your telephone number, and I can see you after we get out?" I had gotten used to the appearance of the women patients, but the men seemed grotesque. I wasn't accustomed to seeing men so helpless or clumsy. Eddie's face was rough with pimples and pustules. In between lumps were pits and craters. To flex that tortured skin into expressions must have been close to painful, but he persisted in raising his eyebrows

34

eagerly, twitching on a smile and blinking as hard as he could. He trembled with eagerness, and I was repulsed by him. Down to essentials here, I was direct. "I can't. I just can't cope with talking to you now."

Eddie nodded. "I know. I'll try again later," he said. I knew he would and I was half grateful. I had let us both down, and I wanted another chance. It wasn't until I was back in the dormitory lying on my bed that I thought about the tone of my answer to him. Although I wasn't very polite, I didn't lie to him. He had responded in kind, and seemed less insulted than pleased that I felt he was worth a straight answer.

Since most of the patients spent the day on the corridor, I had a fair chance of being alone in the dormitory. It happened, however, that in the third bed lay Phoebe, with Evelyn sitting on top of the covers. "Hey, Evelyn," Phoebe was saying, "that was too much, man. Why didn't I think of that earlier?"

"Well, you disappointed me," said Evelyn. "You sure didn't last long." I had climbed onto my bed before I realized what they were talking about. My god, last long at what? and how? I didn't want to hear about it, although the girls didn't seem embarrassed that I was there. They were so casual that, just for a moment, I thought, "All right, you observer, observe! Here's a slice of life for you!" and I did want to hear about it. In any event, there seemed no graceful way to leave.

"I know you," Phoebe was saying, "I bet you've done it with boys."

"I never! Phoebe, you got a dirty mouth. I wouldn't do that with a man. I'm a virgin. I wouldn't never do that before I got married. I am shocked at you, Phoebe!"

"What about that guy you was talking about, that used to take you to the movies?"

"Hell, he just fooled around with me, up in the balcony. I never liked him, and I never let him do what he wanted. I never did do it with him, I promise. I never had a girl, either. You are the only one, Phoebe."

"Well, okay, but don't you let me down. Don't you go messing around with nobody else."

"I wouldn't let nobody eat me but you. But you *are* kind of lazy, Phoebe. I thought you was always telling me what a great lover you are. Look at you, all tuckered out, and we wasn't going at it long at *all*. I could of come four or five more times. You're a pretty poor husband, that's for damn sure."

Oh, what a fraud I was! No observer, I, but on the spot transformed into a Victorian, shocked to my toes. I pored over my paperback but all my conflicting feelings made the type blur on the page. The girls talked on, and I was trapped into bearing witness.

"Well, you just wait. It was because I was nervous, trying to hear if anybody was going to walk in on us. I couldn't have stood it if somebody had walked in on us. Just you wait until we get some privacy sometime, and then I'll show you. I'll eat you up and down."

Evelyn said, "Don't be so mean and mad, Phoebe. We're *married*, now." Phoebe's black hair was stuck to her forehead, and there was a funky sweaty smell in the air. Evelyn laughed, and Phoebe, bashful as a young lover should be, flung a pillow at her.

"Get out of here, and let me sleep. I got to get my strength back, so I can give it to you again."

At the earliest moment I strolled out of the room. I felt shaky. What if I should wake up in the middle of the night to hear them breathing in the next bed, what if I should find them coupled end to end! I was absolutely shocked, yet running alongside these feelings like the second rail on a train's track was shame at my own fears. Why should I care, who had always been so broadminded, who talked tolerance, and always said variety was life's virtue? My first trial, and I was proved a double fraud, not psychotic, but not in control of my feelings, either. And yet I was terrified of those two teen-age girls!

There seemed to be no one I could talk to. As a good patient —and willy-nilly I was turning into a patient in my mind's eye— I should turn to a staff member, perhaps one of the two clinicians on the ward, who functioned as therapists. But then again, neurotic I might be, but not schizophrenic, and I was wary of spending too much time talking to staff. As I stood trembling in the hallway, uncertain of where to turn, another knot inside began to loosen. There was indeed nowhere to go—nowhere to be alone, no one to talk to that was "like me." Like every other patient, I was to be deprived of my privacy for the duration of my stay on N 7, and who was to say that I had more right to object than Phoebe? Certainly Phoebe was unlike any other person on the ward, and lonelier than I; Evelyn must seem little enough comfort, hardly too much for Phoebe to ask for. And yet I could not wrestle down those qualms.

I sought out Miss Sendell in the nurses' office. "I was just wondering if my bed was going to be moved," I said. "After all, it's been in two places so far, and maybe I'm supposed to go somewhere else tonight."

Miss Sendell was mystified. "No, your bed is scheduled to stay where it is. Don't you like that room?"

I hadn't really been intending to tell anyone; in fact, now that I was actually talking to a nurse, I didn't know why I was here. I couldn't expect her to change the way people were made. Moreover, the problem seemed small as I stood in the crowded nurses' office surrounded by women doing the most mundane and matter-of-fact chores, and to complain against another patient seemed a form of treachery. I hated to think of antagonizing Phoebe, and I hated to blame her in front of a nurse.

I ventured, "I think I'm sort of uncomfortable with dykes." Tears came to my eyes and I couldn't control them.

"Oh, heavens. Don't worry about Phoebe. She's very well behaved on the ward. She wouldn't try anything with you." That possibility had not yet occurred to me. "I hope you'll get to like her," Miss Sendell went on. "She and Evelyn are two of the nicest, sweetest girls here. Phoebe has problems, of course. By the way, she's not in here because of the way she organizes her sex life. I think she and Evelyn had something going once; they met in another hospital a long time ago, and this was something of a reunion. Anyway, if anything did start up, we'd know about it, and we'd keep them separate. Don't worry about it. But we can move your bed right now if you want."

"Forget it. It's okay." Sendell was so matter of fact that my reaction seemed hysterical. She didn't know about the "marriage," but I wasn't going to be the one to tell her. My loyalties were realigned once more. Staff didn't have to know everything, not even the nicest nurses, and we patients needed to make our own way. All I had to learn was to be a little more flexible. It was simple. "I'll leave my bed where it is. I'd rather not draw attention to how I was feeling. I guess it was kind of silly." As I walked out I wondered how my record would be reappraised at Bellevue; if Miss Sendell would put a note on my chart under Dr. Sullivan's comments of the night before.

After a macaroni and cheese supper at 5:00 P.M., the television set was turned on and the bridge games took up where they had left off. I practiced being withdrawn. The male patients came to visit again, one of them a tall young Negro with coppery skin and hair arranged in dyed ringlets, elegant as an Egyptian king. Various people said hello to him, and I did, too. He was good-spirited, cheerful, and friendly. "Why, here's a new little one! Aren't you cunning! You can call me Ellis." He had come over to borrow some lipstick. "Hey, Phoebe baby, you are the cutest, sweetest little thing in the world," he said, taking her on his lap. His mascara was neatly in place, his eyebrows plucked, and Rosy Dawn liquid make-up was smeared over his face and neck, and onto his hairless chest. The world had changed so much since the morning that it was natural to see him cradling Phoebe in his arms in a motherly way.

Because this was a Saturday night, the regular night shift was not on duty. The weekend aides were tolerant about our bedtime. Most of the ladies went off to bed of their own accord after medication at 9:00 P.M., but Phoebe and Evelyn stayed up for another hand of bridge with an aide, with Ellis as a fourth, and I spent some time with Miss Rivers, one of the weekend aides. I asked her how long she had worked at Bellevue, and she said it was years.

"But it's changing now, honey, you can see it. It's a regular fancy hotel compared to how it used to be. Why, they used to lock the dormitory during the day so the ladies couldn't lay down if they wanted, they had to be wandering around the hall all the time, and there were just benches to sit on—those chairs there are a new addition. There was a head nurse up here who was a mean old bitch. Oh, I could tell you stories about some of the things that went on here."

"I'd heard some of those stories before I came here. I heard that N 7 was the worst place to be."

"You just forget what you heard, now, you hear? This used to be the violent ward. They used to take all the sick patients from the other wards, when they were *disturbed*, and they'd wrestle them into the elevator and bring them up here. I can remember having to do that many many times. First the jackets, then into the elevator. They didn't have the drugs then that they do now. You can see I'm not built very large myself, and some of those ladies were strong. Sometimes I'd walk around with a mouse under my eye some lady had given me." She chuckled over that.

"But doesn't it ever get to you, particularly late at night? Don't you get depressed?"

"Oh, I keep trying to tell you how much better things are here now. Look at the paint job this place got! Things are changing. They treat the ladies with medication now. They're starting group meetings on some floors—I don't go along with all of that, though. Nobody in their right mind would talk up at one of them." She looked at me askance. "No matter, though. I suppose it's just that way on some of the floors."

"I sort of wondered why I was here, though, on the violent ward. I wondered if they figured I was really crazy, and put me in the worst place."

"It must have been just luck. When did you come up here—Friday? They must have sent a lot of ladies home, and had some empty beds. I was looking around when I came on tonight, and a lot of faces are new here; you aren't the only one. They don't isolate the disturbed ladies any more. When a lady comes in, she goes wherever there's a bed. Too many disturbed ladies together tend to stir each other up, but if you put one or two on a quiet ward, they calm down faster.

"I don't get depressed. I like being with people. Why should I get more miserable here than out on the street? I run into worse outside in the street, any day." She chuckled again. "Darling, today it's you in here, tomorrow it might be me. It don't make a bit of difference."

"But look at us! You can't tell me this isn't a funny crowd to hang around with." I gestured around the corridor. Miss Hargins was nattering to herself in the corner, another lady was hugging her knees and rocking back and forth, back and forth, like an overblown fetus. Someone was banging her head against the wall over and over again.

Miss Rivers said, "Some ladies here are sicker than others. Some need a little bit of time. A few, now, aren't up to much, but most are just like anybody else, except for some little problem. You watch, now: in a couple of days, that lady won't be beating her head that way, and she'll start talking, and you wouldn't know she'd ever been so sick. I suppose you've got some problems, but that don't mean we can't have a nice talk. I got problems, too. There's no guarantee I won't be right in your bed tomorrow, and you back out in the street. I've lived a long, long time, and I know what I'm talking about."

"I trust you, I really do. That's what's crazy—me, a patient, sitting here, and you talking to me as if we have so much in common, and yet you're an aide, and yet you're so different from some of the other aides, and some of the nurses. The crazy thing is that you should be the head nurse or a doctor here, and not an aide on the weekend shift when not so many patients get a chance to talk to you."

"Bless you, honey, but everybody's got a different job to do. They move me around, I'm here, there, wherever they want to put me. Anywhere you go, there's a job to be done."

Miss Rivers hadn't mentioned going to bed, but the head nurse on duty happened to look at the clock, and broke up the bridge game. My last survey of the ward showed two aides moving in on Miss Hargins. "Time for bed, put that away now," they said, as they prepared to carry her down the hall if she put up resistance. She had pulled out a pile of her stolen bread and butter and was gnawing it in the corner like an ancient rat. "Time for bread, time for bread," she said. Luisa strolled down the hall and blew me kisses. I kissed her like a sister, and went to my room. This second night, I slept through to the dawn without waking.

Three

The second day was Sunday. Evelyn had not, after all, paid a midnight visit to Phoebe's bed, and during the night I had heard nothing but her gentle breathing, and snores from Norma June, who was bound to make noise even when she was asleep. When the aide yelled us awake, I stole an extra few minutes in bed, to arrange my mind for the day. In that borderland just the other side of sleep, before I was on my feet and working my way into my bathrobe, lay a sinking feeling that something was very different about this particular day. Something was wrong with it.

It was close to breakfast time before I realized that the snow was still falling outside. I had barely noticed it the day before (we were insulated from weather behind the thick walls), but now, waiting in line for a toilet, I looked out the window into the alley below and saw piles of snow over the pavement and the puddles. Without order in our own minds, our routine was dependent on the stability of the outside to an extent I had not thought much about before. Like the rest of the ladies, I had taken it for granted, like some vast unseen machinery whose breakdown now became apparent only by the absence of its humming. The morning shift had been unable to get to work at all, and so the nighttime aides stayed through the day. The ward, always understaffed on weekends, was now short a couple of nurses.

During the wait for breakfast the chairs were once again arranged in a circle in the corridor, as if we were about to begin playing a parlor game without a leader. Norma June took up her patrol. She beckoned to the girl I had first seen lying on the bathroom floor. "Priscilla, you come over here. You have to learn how to take care of yourself. You have to brush your hair and make yourself look pretty." Priscilla stared into space with a half smile on her lips, and I couldn't tell if she heard Norma June's voice or not. She followed Norma June as docilely as a dog.

By now I had gotten my bearings here among the patients. The ward was becoming familiar. I no longer jumped when Norma June's voice cut through the chatter of the ward like a siren; I scarcely looked up when Luisa began hopping backward down the hall on one foot, chewing her pigtail. The outside world was silent. The snow not only stopped traffic, it muffled the sound of pedestrians struggling down the street. We caught this silent mood on N 7; the patients were subdued. Or perhaps it was only my mood, as I slipped into my periods of "withdrawal" like an old-timer. There were few surprises to look forward to today: the first exhilaration of actually getting in had faded along with the effects of the Dexedrine.

I took my medication obediently, but tucked the Thorazine tablet under my tongue when I drank the paper cup of water. It was easy enough to amble down the hall to the bathroom and drop it in the toilet. I was shaking all over, for it was too easy. Surely someone had seen me, and even another patient

43

might mention it to a nurse. But no, I scanned the faces of the patients I had passed, and no one had paid any attention. I wondered why others didn't dispose of their medication in just this way, and gave a little chuckle of surprise—of course, some did. Most of us were dull-eyed and slow much of the time, but some of the ladies never seemed less than alert. I thought I could pick out those patients by their behavior, and sure enough, I often tended to run into the same women coming out of the bathroom shortly after the medication was doled out.

After breakfast I sat with the others in the corridor and waited for the few diversions offered by a typical Sunday. Because of the blizzard, the usual Protestant church service on the ward had been canceled, and even the Catholic priest didn't arrive until late afternoon. The quiet was broken by the whine of a fat girl named Flo begging an aide for food. "I want to eat! What time is it? Isn't it time for dinner? I want to eat. I'm a growing girl, and I want to eat." Flo wasn't a growing girl, she was thirty or thirty-five, but growing fatter. Her face was long in the chin and slack-jawed beneath small brown eyes. She asked me, "You got anything to eat? Feed a growing girl." She looked like a child wheedling its mother. Norma June often tried to teach her things, for Norma June liked to instruct. She was taller than Flo by a head, and might have weighed fifty pounds less; she was all stringy tendons and long bone, like a Grant Wood pioneer wife, practical at doing chores.

Flo put her plump hand on my knee. "You look like you don't feel good. Have you ever been in Rockland? That's much worse than here. There isn't anything to do there. You're going to like it better here than at Rockland. What do you think of Metropolitan? I think that's the best. What? You've never been in a hospital before! I've been in lots of them. Don't worry, after you get out, you'll get back in again." She patted me to reassure me, and her hand felt like a fat sponge.

During the morning a card game picked up again. Phoebe and Evelyn were quarreling. "I ain't talkin' to you, Phoebe! I'm just going to sit right here and play my hand. You want to go off and cry, you just do it. I won't pay no mind to you."

44

"I wouldn't cry for you, bitch," Phoebe said. Her face looked cold as a Mafia mobster's just before the kill. Then, in a voice soft with self-pity, "You like to hurt my feelings."

"Two hearts. You know I like you a lot, Phoebe, so just you stop being so silly. You always getting your feelings hurt, and I just can't figure it out. Maybe that's your way of getting your kicks."

I went back to my room to be alone for a while, but Norma June and Flo followed me. I was beginning to be able to gauge Norma June's mood by the clock. The nine o'clock medication had almost worn off; there was still an hour to go before the lunchtime medication, and she was agitated. Norma June said, "Do you watch TV? I watch it all the time when I'm at home. I like *Dating Game*, and I like all the quiz shows. My husband and I watch *Dating Game* every time it's on. I heard that when they win that trip to Las Vegas, they don't let them get away with anything. They keep an eye on them all the time, and they don't even get a chance to be alone together. Isn't that something! I'd have to be careful in Las Vegas because I would gamble everything. You have to be careful. You know, some people gamble like it's a disease. There was some people on my block who lost everything they owned. It wasn't from gambling—his partner drank too much. But it's the same thing. People get in so much trouble these days. Do you like *Dating Game* better than the *Newlywed Game?*" She filled me in on the last several installments of *As the World Turns*, and told me I could watch it here.

What inanities! I saw days and days of such conversations stretching ahead of me with no relief. Here was a purgatory to cure me of my sins—deception, fraud, and arrogance, start to finish, would be punished by the most oppressive boredom. I had steeled myself against fear and rage, but boredom like this I had been unable to foresee, I hadn't come close. Norma June said, "My husband—I love my husband, he's wonderful to me, he's so understanding—my husband brought me some bubble gum. I like Dubble Bubble best, don't you? It's the best kind, it never gets hard, no matter how long you chew it. But you know, they don't sell it all over, you've got to look for it. My husband is so wonderful, he hunts all over town for it. Take some."

I said, "Gee, I really don't chew much bubble gum, and that looks like your last piece. Why don't you keep it?"

"No, I want you to have it. It means a lot to me that you take it. You don't have to chew it now, you can save it for a while. But I want you to take it."

Her long fingers twisted the little paper bag nervously. "Please, you've got to. See, I've got some Life Savers, too, and some Bit o' Honeys, but the bubble gum's the best. Take it." She was almost crying. "The doctor says I mustn't give away everything, but I want to, I have to, and I want you to have this. I really tried to be good and I didn't give away more than one or two pieces this morning."

She was so upset, I made a deal with her. "Look, I'll take this piece, but if I don't get around to chewing it this morning, and you feel like you want it, I'll give it back to you later."

"Okay, but I really want you to have it." She looked relieved.

Flo didn't want to be left out. "Here, take this sugar," she said, reaching into her bathrobe pocket for a handful of paper packets taken from the breakfast table.

"No, really, I don't eat much sugar."

Her anxious little eyes took in my hesitation, and she faltered. If conversation was currency, this talk was small change, but when I was least prepared for it, I would be touched by some generous gesture of special value.

"But I want to give you something. I haven't got anything else. I don't have any money to give you. I want to be your friend." She was mortally afraid of being rebuffed or laughed at. I could see that on her face, but she held out the packets to me anyway. Had we been filmed as we spoke, and shown silently on a screen with the tedium of our conversation turned off, we would have looked like serious people who cared about one another. Our faces (even mine) showed concern and attention. Emotions were traded back and forth here more openly than in the real world.

46

"Thank you for the sugar." I put it carefully in my pocket along with my change purse and the piece of bubble gum.

Flo beamed. "I went over to see the boys last night. They always come over here, but nobody ever goes over there, so I did. I wish I had a boy friend. They had a radio going over there, and I danced with them, but they made me leave."

Norma June said, "I heard about you. You were a bad girl, and you should be ashamed of yourself, carrying on like that."

"Can I help it if I have a beautiful body? I just wanted to make the boys happy, that's all. They kept laughing and cheering. They were cheering for *me*, just for me, and I kept dancing and dancing. It's because I have this beautiful body." She began a lumbering waltz in the narrow space at the foot of the beds. "This is what I did last night. They kept clapping and telling me I was such a good dancer and had such a beautiful body. Laughing and clapping—" She flung open her bathrobe and lifted her nightgown up in front of her face. "I'm thirty-six, single, and don't have a man!" Her mountainous white shoulders sloped down from an early widow's hump, and her breasts sagged like giant pears over her huge smooth globular belly. It was solid, round as a beach ball, and the gleaming flesh spread without a wrinkle over its bulk. In the cramped area in which she danced, that belly undulated two feet from my face. I didn't know if it was beautiful, but it was astonishing.

Norma June didn't break stride. "Put down that nightgown. Don't be a bad girl. You know you shouldn't show everything you got. No wonder they kicked you off the men's side last night. You've got to learn some shame."

When I returned with clean sheets from the cart, my bed had been moved again. I didn't know why, or who had given the order. Today was Miss Sendell's day off, and so I couldn't ask her if this was her idea. It seemed best to find my bed as quickly and quietly as I could, and not draw attention to its new location. I found it in one of the two large dormitory rooms; here, in a space some twelve feet by twenty, were fourteen beds squeezed in end to end, and with barely room at each side to tuck in the covers. I was glad to be with more patients; I wanted to get to know as many as I could. At the head of my bed was Evelyn's, at the foot, Priscilla's. There was so little space that Gerta's bed stuck out halfway into the corridor.

Before lunch I saw Mrs. Briggs, the grieving woman who was so concerned for me my first day on the ward. She seemed to be waiting by the dining-room door for someone to talk to her, and I obliged by asking her how she was feeling. "I'm trying to decide whether to go in there," she said. She nodded toward the dining room. "I haven't been eating very well. I haven't been taking my meals with the people in there; they've been bringing food to my room. I don't think I'm very hungry." Like the other patients I tended to disregard words. I picked up my cue from the supplication in her eyes. When the nurse's aide bellowed, "Dinner, ladies!" I put my arm around Mrs. Briggs and walked her in to sit at a table. She took tentative, trembling steps, and leaned against me for support as if she were an old woman. We had a special Sunday dinner of chicken and peas and mashed potatoes, with ice cream for dessert. Mrs. Briggs ate like a starving refugee.

The social worker arrived late, shaking the snow off her boots. On the weekends there was just one, who worked part time. She was tiny and had wispy long hair. She asked to speak to me, and I was nervous about the meeting. I took a seat in the office, and she sat at one of the big wooden desks. She looked like a college girl, and when I asked her, she admitted she was going to St. John's. She was very serious. I had noticed that the staff members tended to be serious in proportion to the importance of their jobs. The doctors were the most serious of all, but some of the aides were whimsical. This girl may have been trying to make up for her youth with her professional manner; indeed, she sobered me, and I called her Miss Garber, although I figured I had an easy ten years on her.

I told her in a small voice that I didn't have a job, that I didn't want to go into details about it, I just didn't, but I wasn't working now. I let her pull each piece of information out of me, question by question, because I thought a patient in this predicament probably would not be ready to open up so quickly, and to this young girl. In fact I didn't want her to know anything about me. She put out a few feelers about what would happen when I got out of the hospital.

"What kind of job do you think you would like?" she asked. I had told her that I was unable to get enough work as a free-lance editor to support myself. "You be thinking about what to do, and come to talk to me at any time. We ought to be able to help you find a job where you'll be happy—maybe something like a clerk or a typist."

I responded without thinking. "If I'm going to get a job, I should think it should be one I'm going to last at. I'd be bored to tears shuffling file folders." I was irritated that she assumed I was suited for dull jobs she wouldn't dream of taking for herself. She jumped as if she saw me plainer than I meant her to, and I realized my error. Presumably I had failed at my editorial work because I couldn't take the pressure and the responsibility. Recently discharged patients doubtless settled down gratefully to jobs they might be technically overqualified for, just because the jobs were routine, and easier to succeed at. No wonder Miss Garber was used to suggesting jobs as a dishwasher or sewing-machine operator or assembly-line worker to patients I often found particularly quick-witted. A few of the patients were so kind and commonsensical they might take over Miss Garber's job and show a flair for it. So I quickly backtracked, and mumbled that I really didn't know what I wanted to do, and I would think it over.

"I see you have a friend here in the city," Miss Garber said, checking the chart. "I wish you'd ask her to come in to talk to the social worker. It will be Miss Nichols or Miss Roy during the week. I know either one would like to talk to her. In the meantime, I'll try to reach her this afternoon."

I left the office wondering if I had gotten in over my head. I appreciated the efforts the hospital was making for me, but they were much more thorough than I had thought likely, and poor Helen was going to be called upon to do more acting than either of us had planned.

Back in the hallway, someone said to me, "I think the sun is shining."

"I hope it is," I said. The snow was still falling.

"I think it is. I'm trying to get better. You should have seen me when I came in here. Boy, was I sick!" She made a disgusted wave of her hand, and laughed. She was eighteen, and a schizophrenic. I hadn't spoken to her before, but I had watched her often. There was something fey and graceful about her that was immensely appealing. Her hair was extraordinary colors: black at the roots, then bright yellow for three or four inches, then orange-red to the ends; she looked like some animal in the woods wearing protective coloring. Her eyes were huge and protuberant; she carried her head slightly forward, her chin raised up, as if looking out for danger. She picked her way through the ward like a fawn through underbrush, but when she spoke she was all Brooklyn, tough and adenoidal. "I get so mixed up sometimes, you know, when I don't concentrate. I've got to keep my mind on things, or else I get sick again. I think I trust people too much. The doctor says I trust people too much. I have to concentrate on being holy."

I said, "I don't know about being holy. I'd be satisfied with getting well."

"The doctor's pretty nice. I don't know, though, I think she doesn't think I'm so good. The people sometimes get on my nerves, I don't like them near me. They're dirty, you know?"

I said, "We all have to take a shower every day."

"I mean dirty inside. Crummy. Sometimes people are, you know, they don't care about you. I was walking around this room in my head. It was underground, like a church, with pretty windows. I was all by myself, inside my head, and there were these big pillars, and it was all stone. I liked it, all right. Now you see why you've got to be holy." She nodded her head as if everything was explained. I asked her name; it was Jeannette Rosetti, and she had been in several hospitals before. I seemed to be one of the very few patients who was not a veteran of at least two previous hospital visits. "I'm going to leave here pretty soon; they're going to send me home because I'm not sick any more," Jeannette said cheerfully.

The twelve o'clock medication had been the same dose of Thorazine, but in liquid form, and I had seen no way to avoid swallowing it. It tasted terrible, and puckered the tongue. "That tastes so bad," I said. "Can't I have a pill instead?"

"Not on your life," the nurse said. She looked me straight in the eye and I wondered if she knew I didn't take the pills. In the little paper cups I saw that some of the patients on Thorazine had pills waiting for them. I looked as innocent as I could. My only hope was that the other nurses were not so clever; this nurse was one of the night nurses, weaving on her feet from tiredness, and I didn't want to give her any trouble.

I knew how the drug worked by now. I had about twenty minutes of a gradually intensifying and fairly pleasant high still ahead of me, and then I would start to get groggy. There would be no way out of taking a nap. During the high my mind would float off on tangents. Before it put me to sleep I wanted to plot out my meeting with the doctor the next day, although I knew that I could hardly plan for it realistically without knowing what he was like or the pattern of questions he would ask. When I tried to picture him, his age, his manner, my mind went blank. If he was like Dr. Sullivan I wouldn't like him at all, but any happier alternative I couldn't imagine. If I gave him a face in my mind, I ran some risk. If he was a real person to me, I would not dare to meet him at all. It was easier to think of him as a function of hospital life, something mechanical. Like an addict heading for his heroin I was drawn to fruitless planning of conversations and tactics. If I said one thing, he would respond thus; if I tried a different approach, he would surely go another way. I let myself assume him to be just as trusting as the social worker. He would probably see me once to take my history, he would see me a second time to note my improvement and consider releasing me, if I played my cards right, and then a third time to be sure that I was quite well, and shortly thereafter he would sign the release papers. I asked an aide when I would see the doctor, and she told me I was down for Mondays and Thursdays. By any arithmetic, I should be in the hospital a week and a half, or perhaps two weeks, at the minimum. I had to think of some way to get out in seven days; I had no choice about that. Each day in the hospital was costing me close to a hundred dollars, which I was bound to pay, and I had hardly enough money in the bank to cover a week. Each patient here paid according to ability, and as I was not on welfare, I reckoned I must pay the entire bill. I might get in a good deal of trouble if I tried to fool Blue Cross into helping me. I could see myself headed for jail for fraud or theft of services. Looking around at the other patients, I figured I might be the only lady here to pay the full rate, and pay it by herself.

But my mind kept losing track of these practicalities and winging off into fantasies of being discovered, or shipped off to a state hospital by mistake, or being kept here for months. I tried to fend off sleep, but I seemed to dream with my eyes open. I knew how easily one could slip into mild paranoia here, yet I couldn't assess the extent of that paranoia, or the extent to which fears were justified. I could trust no guide here except the balance inside myself, but maybe the atmosphere in this ward had worked its way through my psyche like smoke seeking out the cracks in a brick wall, and I had lost my perspective without knowing it.

Then, like a pendulum, I would swing off in the other extreme. Perhaps I was not acting sick enough! Anyone watching me answering questions, brushing my teeth, eating my food neatly, might conclude I was functioning again, and release me. The doctor might say on Monday, "You are much better, Miss Barry. You may leave today." After all, I couldn't think of a single psychotic symptom I'd shown since I came in here. I was obviously neither homicidal nor suicidal, and if I showed neither of these tendencies, the law encouraged the hospital to release me.

But by now Helen might have talked to the social worker, and I might be able to pick up a clue from her. I waited in line for the telephone, letting everyone else go first so I might have a better chance of being alone when my turn came. It was almost 3:00 when I had the telephone to myself. (I stole privacy like a thief.) I asked Helen if they thought me very sick, or well. Should I start hinting at my "secret plan" for evading the man who was following me? Should I admit to a depression, and invent dreams of coffins and bottles of poison? "For God's sake, no," Helen said. "You're in. You're really in. Now we must start working on some way to get you out."

I fell asleep as soon as I stretched out on my bed, for once again the ward was stifling hot. An hour later I woke up with a headache that began at the base of the skull and worked its way over both temples, a whining kind of pain that scattered my thoughts, the fruit of that hothouse sleep. When I asked Miss Sendell for an aspirin, she said she would have to get a special order from the doctor, and this might take time. There was only one doctor on duty on Sundays for all the wards in the psychiatric building.

"I'm not looking for cocaine, methedrine, or bennies. All I want is an aspirin. It's not even a prescription drug." No, impossible. Against all regulations. "I'll bet you have one in your pocketbook, Miss Sendell. God, I'd be willing to pay. Think of the extra income. You could peddle them on the side."

I fell into a sour and imperious mood. Such concern for the patients' health—I should be grateful! Caught here with the steam heat hissing, sweating as the temperature passed eighty, all the windows sealed tight against the snow, surrounded by thirty-odd women with foul breath and damp armpits, I was in a cage that had no bars to rattle or beat against. The Thorazine had worn off. Now I knew why so many patients took it without question; under drugs a slow shuffle down the corridor sufficed, but let us out from under tranquilizers, and the need for exercise surfaced. Hunger, sex, exhaustion—these were nothing to the frustration of being unable to move freely. I would have organized calisthenics or a relay race on the spot, except for the heavy traffic in the corridor. I imagined Team One (the retarded, the paranoid, the delusional) pulling ahead of Team Two (the abstracted, the lobotomized, the phobic) while the

53

aides cheered them on, only to lose out on penalties for mowing down the senile, the catatonic, and the physically infirm, who refused to participate, and blocked the hall. I was desperate for motion. I dreamed of playing tennis on a court near an ocean breeze, of riding a roller coaster or climbing a mountain. I thought of silence and wind. Here was always the scurrying of women, scraps of half-heard conversations, whispers, sighs, mutters, dead air. For the young and the healthy, it was like being shut in a coffin. The nurses, who could close the door to their office or take a coffee break off the ward, who ate their lunch far from our clattering tables, should expect headaches in those penned here and hand us a bottle of aspirin with our hospital gown, to take at our discretion.

I waited in silent rebellion for word from the doctor, and it never came. Did the message get through to him? Did his reply get passed back? I never knew. What was more painful than the headache was the dependence. Not to be able to take an aspirin on my own was to be treated like a child, and I reacted like a child. I was sullen, and more angry than I should have been. When I was eight or nine I plotted running away from home, and packed up a lunch. Here, totally unaware of the parallel, I worked out escapes. It was the next best thing to running away. Resentfully I worked out the logistics of my release. I responded as if to a personal challenge. I might not be able to cadge an aspirin, but I would plot my moves for the next week with the skill of an international spy. Because children are weak and small, their instincts for survival are finally attuned, and becoming a child in my mind made me shrewd and gave me satisfaction.

If I was correct in figuring that the doctor would wish to see me twice after the worst of my "illness" was over, I should appear to be already on the road to recovery when I met him for the first time on Monday. Even if I seemed quite well, the doctor would probably wish to talk to me on Thursday to make sure my improvement was continuing at a good pace, and at that time he might authorize my release on Friday or Saturday.

I tried to think of some way to make Monday's mental health

credible. There should be some sort of transitional act to show I was coming around. I remembered the letter to Mayor Lindsay that I had retrieved from the police, and again from the aide who issued me my nightgown and slippers. I took it out of hiding from between the pages of my paperback book, and waited until the social worker was alone in her office.

"You said I might talk to you if I wanted to," I said.

"Come right in. What would you like to talk about?" She was wearing a green shirt and a short grey skirt. Her legs were thin, and her knees a little bumpy. She folded her hands over them. "What's on your mind, Miss Barry?"

In my baggy nightgown, my hair straggling down my back uncurled and unbrushed, no lipstick, I felt at a disadvantage with this neat young girl, but she owned me here, she was staff. And I had to call her Miss Garber, not Joan, and she had to call me Miss Barry, as if we were equals, and we were not. I wished we could call each other by first names, but was ashamed to ask her to. Her face was composed as carefully as if she had aligned the muscles with her fingers: this face would not show shock, or fear, or laughter, no matter what I did. She was prepared for anything. I might act arbitrary, illogical, withdrawn, sly, or wheedling, with only partial or sporadic use of reason.

At the same time, I felt another pressure, a pressure from back on the corridor, a sort of practical rule of thumb passed without words from old patient to new, and, quite unwittingly, from kind staff members such as this young social worker. "If you want to get out, act right. You don't have to know why you're supposed to come on in a certain way, or even how, but look sharp, pick up the clues," this wisdom said. From staff I soon learned that I should try to be good, co-operative, respectful. I must appear serious about wanting to get well. My psyche was humming like a tuning fork, picking up alternating appeals to total freedom and careful control, and standing in the doorway I tingled with a special sort of exhilaration I was to feel again and again. To be so free! To be able to talk nonsense, or insult anyone I disliked! And yet, be careful! Hold back!

55

"I wrote a letter," I said, and stopped as if I couldn't go on. "It's hard for me to talk about it."

Miss Garber would put no pressure on me. "Perhaps you'd like to think about talking about it for a while. I'll be here all day, and you can talk about it later."

"No, no—you see, I—well, it's got to be done now. It didn't come out right, the letter, I mean. It's—it isn't a good letter. Something is wrong with it. I don't know what's wrong with it; I don't know how I'd write it differently right now." I started to hold out the letter.

Miss Garber didn't move. "Why is it so hard for you to talk about it?" She was opening negotiations by small steps of logic. With a sick person, you don't say: Give me the letter and I'll tell you what I think of it. Miss Garber said, "If you don't want to give it to me, you don't have to."

"Do you talk to the doctor?" I asked. "Do you tell him everything I say?" I knew there wasn't a chance Miss Garber would keep this conversation to herself, and it would not serve my purpose if she did so, but at the same time I wanted her to say no. The staff was in conspiracy, it seemed to me from the other side, they would talk about me, and I couldn't control what they would say. Miss Garber hedged. "I can tell the doctor if you'd like me to," she said, as if I could make the choice.

"I wrote this letter to Mayor Lindsay," I said. "I was trying to say something but this doesn't say it right. I don't think the doctor should see it. I'm afraid if the doctor sees it—" My chin began to tremble, and to my astonishment, tears started to roll down my face.

Miss Garber looked at my face with the same tranquil seriousness, as if listening to my expressions rather than watching them, and as if she couldn't see the tears at all. I was a specimen being studied by an attentive laboratory technician. I was coming apart completely. I was angry and embarrassed, so I leaped to my feet, flung the letter on the desk, and ran out of the office.

In the bathroom I splashed water on my face. The other patients had not noticed my tears, or at least made no comment about them. People often behave peculiarly in Bellevue, and a few tears are common enough. Tears yesterday with Miss Sendell, tears today with Miss Garber—for no reason at all. In the scratched metal mirror my face looked pale and frightened and I almost didn't recognize myself. The outlines were blurred. I couldn't decide whether the Bellevue atmosphere was making me odder than I was outside, or whether it was bringing to the surface some instability that had never been tested in the outside world. I hurried back to the corridor, and chose a chair behind the open door of the social workers' office. I placed my chair so that I could see through the crack between the hinges. Miss Garber could not see me. She was reading intently, her shoes neatly parallel, with the same precise expression on her face. She took a long time with my letter; she must have read it ten times. Some aides went into the office for their break, and the door was closed.

Luisa was singing a song to herself. A new patient had arrived, a little mole of a woman, white, with white hair, and her face collapsed around her toothless mouth. Luisa moved toward her as if pulled by a witch's spell. The little old lady's eyes peeped out, suspicious, shrewd. Luisa's eyes did not focus, she did not look at the woman, but her body seemed to find her on its own. Like a huge fish Luisa flopped on her, arms as limp as flippers, a dead weight. Then one of her hands reached into the frizzy white hair and pulled slowly and deliberately. The old woman gurgled back in her throat, and her terrified scream sounded like a squawk. It took two aides and two patients to pull Luisa away. "Padre, padre," Luisa said as they took her down the hall to seclusion, "padre, padre."

Priscilla, oblivious to this scene, asked the new patient, "Cigwette? Cigwette?" her only word. For the last few hours she had been plucking butts from ashtrays and from the floor. Priscilla's fingers were stained brown. Cigarettes were the only thing that brought animation to her face. "Cigwette? Cigwette?" Up and down the ward she moved, a busy panhandler. The new little lady drew away from her in disgust. There was something about this patient that I didn't very much like, and

I couldn't tell what it was. I had not spoken a word to her, nor had I heard her speak to anyone else, but I felt no urge to be friendly or to reassure her. I wondered if Luisa in some way had picked up the same response to her.

After supper my headache faded at last of its own accord. A woman from Jamaica struck up a conversation with me. "How do you like this place?" she asked. "I think it stinks pretty much. I commit myself, my husband bring me here, because I am a addict, but I want to get out of this place. They don't do nothing for you here if you are a addict." Her thin face made a tight triangle; she would have been pretty had not her cheeks looked hollow, and her skin ashy under the brown. "Last time I was on the fourth floor, but this time they put me up here, like I'm a crazy person. I don't know why they do this to me. Last time they give me some good medicine, this time they don't give me nothing. This city is a bunch of shit. There is no help here. For a addict, you have to go into the hospital, but they don't want you. So you got to make some doctor say you are crazy, just to get you in. They know you are here because you are a addict, but they don't treat you different. They don't do nothing for what is killing you, they watch you suffer."

I liked talking to her because there was no translation problem. With Priscilla or Luisa or Jeannette I could figure out where any given conversation was headed, but the vocabulary of schizophrenics was an odd one, made up of metaphor, silences, non sequiturs, head-shakings, gestures with the hands, grunts— we seemed to understand one another, but it was a pleasant change to have a talk in English. Selina, the addict, said, "I hear you was asking the nurse for a aspirin. You are pretty dumb. You know those fucks, they won't give you nothing simple like that. You get your friends to bring you some."

"If somebody brings in pills from the outside, can't they get caught at it? I'm in enough trouble already, just being here."

"Oh, you are so dumb, you little one. They don't check nothing. You get your friends to bring in aspirin, anything you want. My husband, the last time, he brought me in drugs when I asked him. I take Seconal, and he bring me in all the pills I want, and I take them right on the ward." I didn't ask her why she bothered to come into the hospital if she was going to take drugs here, too, but she answered anyway. "I didn't like it here. I got a little better. Then I give in to myself. So what the hell, every addict does this, you watch after visiting hours, you look at the addicts, and you see everybody high." Selina said that the only exception to this pattern was on the fourth floor, where a very few patients were given methadone in an experimental program. "I came in here thinking I could get that," she said. "I always have bad luck. I come here five days ago, and the doctor looks at me for five minutes only, and I haven't seen anyone since then. If I don't see a doctor soon, I'm going to ask my husband to take me out of this place. It's just for crazy people here."

After dinner I flipped through an old *Ladies' Home Journal* I found under the wooden bench in the corridor. The cover was ripped off and it was four months old. I counted the number of times my eye caught phrases like: mental health, emotional sickness, neurotic symptom. I skimmed rather than read, and found fourteen such references, including one cartoon and two one-line comments from the "Poor Woman's Almanac."

The card game began: Evelyn, Phoebe, Sally Rinzler, an aide named Miss Kearnes. All, as they talked over the cards, healthy. Normal. No kooks here. Sally, in fact, was almost ready to go home. She was dark and looked like a pretty, quiet college student. She didn't talk much to us new or eccentric patients; not that she was unfriendly, but her mind was on other things, she was looking toward the end of the week and her release. She was one of the few who read novels from the hospital library, and she talked only to the most lucid patients, or spent her time by herself.

When Miss Kearnes or Ellis did not make a fourth, that seat was taken by Eileen Thibeau, another teen-ager, with pink cheeks and eyes made up like a movie star. These "normal" patients got along particularly well with the aides, for they were no trouble. Except when Phoebe lost her temper or Evelyn shortsheeted Eileen's bed or started a pillow fight, they were easy to be with. Each of these girls had been here a long time.

At 7:00 P.M., Eileen yelled out, "Snack bar!" Had I entered the building last Friday by the front door, I might have noticed the small counter off the lobby where the aides picked up sandwiches and Cokes for lunch, and where certain patients with this special privilege waited in a long line of sagging bathrobes and floppy slippers. Eileen cherished this job; and two or three times a day she yelled out with the authority of the toughest aide, and collected orders. She was smart. She took the money in advance, and she shut some people off. Always a crowd collected before her expeditions. To Flo she was kind: "No, I can't get you a jelly donut, because you don't have any money. Every time, you ask me; and every time, I tell you no. How am I going to get you food with no money? The man will laugh at me."

"Somebody give me a penny, give me a nickel, somebody, for a growing girl. Is a penny enough?"

To some Eileen was harsh. "You, Hargins, shut up. Get away."

"Oh, watch your step, young lady, or I'll tell the Governor about you, you know what we do to people like you, who won't shut up, we lock you up, we throw away the key!" She babbled in her singsong until Eileen stamped her foot and said, "*Jesus*, get her out of here, Miss Pinero!"

"Watch your step! Does the Governor know? Albany is very close to here, twenty-five miles as the crow flies, do we think we're crazy? Throw away the key! Shut up, shut up! Give me some smokes, folks? Jelly, ha, ha, eat your nose, donut, all the way to Albany! The architect, he'll lock you up! Just ask my brother, thank you, Governor, don't be a silly donut!"

"Go comb your hair," Phoebe said.

Warily Miss Hargins pulled her fingers through that spiky fluff, and it instantly eased up on end again. "Oh, go to Albany, Governor!" the tiny nasal voice wore on like a dentist's drill.

Miss Kearnes bullied us jovially into bed later. While the corridor light was still as bright as its limited wattage would allow, before Miss Kearnes came around for the nightly bed check, I made a few more notes in the margins of my book. The conversations I had overheard had the cockeyed logic of nursery rhymes.

During this day I had run through irritation, nervousness, boredom; the small emotions, nothing heroic, nothing important. All around me, the worst sort of tragedy—battered psyches, broken-down minds—and yet we fell into routines and rituals here, jokes, the exchange of information, as if this were an ordinary sort of world, demanding no more of us than the most petty response. What made the inmates here turn away from their old lives like old clothes that no longer fit; what made them discard family, friends, work, all ordinary purpose? Or what made them believe this place was refuge?

I had looked to discover revelation here, but the moments were rare, and they were fleeting. An embrace, a smile, the clutch of a hand, the effect passing as quickly as a breeze turning over the leaves of a tree; no more than one found outside these walls. Just as outside, one had to settle for what one could get. Yet in those moments when the truth broke through, if only we were grand enough for the occasion, no doubt we should profit. But we are querulous and small, and when God himself shook a soul loose among us, we turned our backs, we relentlessly adjusted. We found our health in banality.

I tucked my book under my pillow as Miss Kearnes loomed against the light. Her face fell in shadow; she was a blunt square shape with no features. "Jenks, Rosetti, Rinzler, Barry, Foster, Nieves," she said, ticking off the names on the clipboard in her hand. The rest of the list blended with fragments of dreams, the sour smell of urine from someone's bed, and from another bed, a rhythmic creak like a squeaky wheel. Somewhere nearby lay a bed-wetter, and somewhere someone's sweaty palms jerked at the metal bars of the bedframe. It was all the same to me.

Four

My dream was set in a drawing room. Ladies passed through the French doors wearing long satin dresses with tight bodices and bustles. The scent of lilacs drifted in the open windows, and a girl was sitting at the harpsichord, striking the keys with her long white fingers. The mood was serene; the stage was set for a comedy of manners. Filtering through the sunbeams came a soft voice, "Get up, sweetheart, you get up now, little Annie. You're almost late for breakfast." One of the ladies had turned from the harpsichord to place her hand on my shoulder, gentle as a dove, but when I looked hard at it, the hand was brown, and it was shaking me awake. Evelyn said, "I let you sleep this time, and you sure are a good sleeper. You didn't hear nothing. You didn't hear Miss Scanlon yellin' at us, you just looked sweet as a baby sleeping there. Now you get up, you hear?"

The plumbing was already clanking and complaining in the bathroom, the radiators were banging, Norma June was herding latecomers to the toilets. I had slept like a private adjusted to the shriek of mortars. The harder the aides yelled each morning, the harder I slept, and for the rest of the week, I relied on Evelyn's gentle voice.

At breakfast, Norma June organized the bowls of cereal that people didn't want to eat and gave them to Flo, who ate three of them, one after another. Today the confrontation with the doctor, and the end to uncertainty. Something was going to move. When I saw the doctor, I might uncover what he thought of madness through how he dealt with it in me. I was so eager for the meeting the adrenalin raced through my system, and I was in a fine mood.

I had intended to stay sober and parsimonious with my feelings at least until after I had seen the doctor, but it had been several days now since I had laughed out loud, or heard a joke, or told a joke, and I missed humor. The aides joked among themselves. I was as yet uncertain how freely we patients might join in. I corked up my natural good spirits from moment to moment, and during the morning shower some worked its way out like bubbles from a stoppered soda bottle. Once again the dreary line of women filed into the shower room, stumbled out of robes and gowns, and under the spray, some half asleep, all dull-faced and shambling. Then, half dry, with goose flesh white or brown or pinkish-beige, taking without a glance the gown the aide held out. Once again Evelyn was helping. "Get moving, ladies," she said. "Step up now and get your dresses." When my turn came, she handed me a brown seersucker robe that came to the floor.

"Evelyn, I won't take it. I want another dress. I want one short enough so you can see my knees."

"But, honey, you're just a shrimp, I bet you ain't five feet tall, and they don't carry your size at this here store."

"Evelyn, I'm telling you, I won't leave until you find me a Paris original in that bin."

Evelyn laughed, the aides laughed, the patients in the

shower were smiling, and some of those who were through with their showers helped Evelyn sort through the big canvas bin. At the very bottom was a flowered gown that was missing its snaps and its sash, but which came only to mid calf. "Straight from Paris for you, darlin'. They call this a maxi," Evelyn said, helping me into it. I posed like a mannequin. The aides clapped and whistled.

"What are you in such a good mood for?" an aide asked me, almost as an afterthought.

"Well, can't a person be in a good mood for no reason?" I asked, wondering if she saw something amiss. At moments like this I never sorted the paranoia from the truth, and perhaps the paranoia was the truth; perhaps in a psychiatric ward, it's healthy to be a little paranoid.

Today the ward was bustling. It was a Monday morning, and enough of the snow was cleared off the streets for the staff to get to work. We ladies, too, had our Monday routine. We prepared to meet with student nurses, clinicians, and doctors. Two or three ladies dressed carefully in street clothes, and left on passes to look for work or apartments. At nine o'clock the student nurses arrived like a flock of busy birds, in stiff white pinafores and blue and white striped blouses. They were all young, fresh-faced, most of them pretty, and every one of them was white. They crowded into the corridor as if this was a classroom just before a study period was called to order; and this was literally true. The student nurses picked up conversations with one patient, then another. We were the lessons for the day. When a patient was willing to talk, they would settle (each nurse like a hen puffing her feathers over a nest, smoothing her skirt under her and arranging the stiff pinafore). A blond nurse was with Priscilla. "Don't you feel like talking today?"

Priscilla said nothing.

"Why don't you want to talk, Priscilla?"

Priscilla looked into space.

"Are you angry at me? We're only trying to help you."

Priscilla smiled to herself.

"Well, if you don't want to talk, I'll come back later," the student nurse said in a businesslike way, and moved on to another patient.

"You came in over the weekend," another nurse said to me. Her hair was soft brown and naturally curly tendrils curled softly out from the net that held it back from her face. Her eyes were blue and widely spaced, her cheeks a fresh pink, and there were freckles on her nose. She was a natural beauty, fresh as new cream. She asked why I was here, and I told her about being in Washington Square Park, and about the two boys that brought me to the police station. I said I guessed I was making a lot of noise. She smiled encouragement and said her name was Miss McMullen.

A ruckus eddied at the other side of the corridor. Alvine Foster had won by good behavior this morning her wig (bright red) and her false teeth, and the freedom of the ward. But now she rose up, tore off her false hair, threw her teeth on the floor. Flexing her arms like a fierce small ape, she swung toward the television set on its stand in the corner. Before anyone thought to stop her, she leaned over, embraced it, and hurled it to the floor. For perhaps thirty seconds the ward hesitated in shock; the only sound was the tinkling of broken parts sifting through the smashed works and onto the floor. Triumphant, Mrs. Foster ripped off her hospital dress, and stood with her chin out, ready to take on the world. What slyness in her eye, what courage against an enemy invisible to us, but there, there before her as surely as she stood there, fists clenched. She smiled a brief welcome to that enemy, an old enemy met a hundred times before, and conquered often as not, in her own battles on a psychic field far from this ward. One could imagine her ancestors incarnate in her now, her gnarled bare feet testing the African savannah, not this shabby brown linoleum; her fist might grasp a spear instead of the antenna of a broken television set.

"OOO-EEE!" she cried out, a grand mad victory cry. "I'se done it now!" And one was tempted to cheer along with her, hooray for power, cheers for destruction and guile. For how stealthily she had crept up to the foe, how rapidly she had shed the trappings of Mrs. Foster the rational, skidded the plastic teeth across the floor, smeared the red lipstick with her hand like blood-red stain. And what freedom! to face the enemy so, naked, plain. Such a tiny woman, ancient, yet quick and smooth-skinned, just a hint of puckering over the belly, the sagging breasts still round, the flesh firm, dents and dimples in the buttocks—she cried out again, "Ooo-eee!" for this was her fine moment, satisfaction close to sexual in its nature, confident and proud, standing still now with both feet planted, waiting for those intruders who immediately clustered around her, pinioned her arms, pulled her back on her heels, swathed her in a robe, expertly jackknifed her knees, slid her into a wheelchair, into the canvas jacket, and down the hall; that victory lost now in less time than it had taken to win it. Mrs. Foster mumbled as they wheeled her away, a complaining explanation that no one could understand. It was in another language, out of this time, spoken by those on the other side who kept silence now as if respecting her privacy, not letting on that they, too, spoke that tongue, they too had relished such triumphs, and ended like her, in confusion, giggling and whining in that rolling chair.

But we picked up our business quickly enough. Such drama was too common to interest us for long. Only Luisa watched Mrs. Foster being wheeled off to seclusion, and then came over to hug me. Today her eyes were in focus, and she searched my face like a blind person just given sight. She seemed quiet, depressed, rational.

"How are you?" she asked in English, with only the most delicate Spanish accent. I asked her if she remembered me from the night we were both admitted. "In the blue room," she said, "in the room with the blue chairs. You were there with the man who was holding you, like so—" she cradled her arms in the air beside her. "How could I ever forget you?" she said.

An hour later Luisa was skipping down the hall again and speaking Spanish. She hummed and swayed over the blocked-up water fountain, and turned the faucet on full, singing a little song as it overflowed onto the floor and splashed on her broad, immobile feet. "No, Luisa," I said, as I helped an aide and another patient pull her away. "Leave the fountain alone." She looked right through me.

Surely, if she so clearly remembered Friday night, she would remember this moment too, and all those other moments she had left our world for her own. I tried to see this scene through her eyes: the cluster of faces close to hers, the voices scolding and cajoling; what did we look like? What did she hear in our voices? I tried to block out words, which clearly she was paying no attention to, and hear tones. The aide with an arm around Luisa's waist was saying, "Let go now, that's a good girl," but there were beads of sweat on her upper lip and with one hand she was struggling to pry Luisa's fist from the faucet. For a few minutes I thought I caught Luisa's double vision, like two movie screens going at once, nonsensical actions superimposed on one another. The grunting aide, the curious and unconcerned eye of a patient, kind words and grimaces, the tightening grip around the waist, finally the modified half nelson that lifted her half into the air; all these images were clear and discrete, yet fit no pattern, each fragment of action a piece of broken time. That's two, I thought, as they emptied a second small room of beds and laid Luisa on the bare floor (she would not stand) and locked the door.

At 10:00 the doctors came onto the ward. One was a woman, quiet and efficient, one was a small harried man. He was pointed out to me as the doctor I was to see in one of the two tiny offices behind the dining room. I had to wait my turn, and many others seemed more anxious than I. Patients clustered around the doctors demanding attention.

Mrs. Briggs yelled, "That doctor should have his license taken away from him. He strongly implied that I was insane. I'm not a lunatic. I didn't try to take my own life, he's not fit to practice. I'd be interested to know his credentials!" Leola Gibson said, "You're right, he's no good for you."

"When am I going to get my operation, doctor?" Sadie Till

said. "I'm hurting so much. I keep thinking it's coming every day, and then it don't come." The doctor nodded his way through the women, murmuring comments to each side, now and again looking at the dining-room door as if gauging the shortest number of steps to reach it.

When my turn came I sat in a chair facing the doctor at his wooden desk. On the wall was a list of psychological disorders: I. Undifferentiated Schizophrenia. II. Paranoia. Et cetera. Et cetera. The doctor was looking through my file folder. Spirited from under the hand of the social worker lay, right on top, the letter to Mayor Lindsay. The doctor saw me look at it and tilted up the corner of the folder.

Dr. Kegan was small, tense, and concerned. His face was narrow, his eyes large and black. A professional schizophrenia had split his face in two: his mouth was expressionless as he read, the mouth of a man who was professionally calm, a properly blank screen, formal, orderly, regular in his habits. It was the mouth of a man of precise attitudes. But above the upper lip, chaos ruled. The eyes protested with tics and twitches, the eyebrows quivered, the nostrils flared. He had a way of lifting his eyebrows at odd moments, as if straining to explore his receding hairline.

We ran through the litany, beginning once again, "Why are you here, Miss Barry?" precisely as before. I sat looking at my hands and trembling lest I be found out, for which should I address, that calm mouth that conjured up a private practice at forty dollars an hour, post-menopausal depressions and anxiety neuroses, or would the eyes find me out? They had learned something, those eyes, picked up mad inspiration from each surrogate Virgin Mary, each intimate to international conspiracy, and all those listeners to secret electrical currents; the eyes acknowledged those voyagers who traveled comfortably in lands without maps, where a fifty-minute hour ticked off on a psychiatrist's clock meant less than ten minutes' talk with the devil.

But to my astonishment he averted those eyes from mine like a man hiding some shameful news; he looked down at his hands, at the floor, in the direction of my ear, around my hairline, the pupils shifting rapidly. We both had secrets, he and I. I thought he might be, simply, sorry for me, and so for himself, and thus he struck this bargain with me: he would not stare me down, and I was to keep my eye focused on his immobile chin. I felt that it was I that had committed the crime he was hiding.

Hoping to hurry us both through this encounter, I suggested that after all, I was feeling ever so much better, and perhaps with Helen's help, and the co-operation of my minister, I might get the promise of a job filing papers in the parish office.

"Not yet, Miss Barry. First we have to find out why you were so upset." We ran through my personal history. "Where were you born?"

"Boston."

"Have you lived in Texas all your life?"

"Texas!"

"Oh, I thought you said Austin," said Dr. Kegan, with something close to a giggle. We continued through my personal history, slipped past my lack of a family, my unstable working career. During a pause in the conversation Dr. Kegan looked into space for a moment, shook his head again, and said to himself, "Boston! Hm-m," as if I weren't there at all.

He was nonplused and quirky, and I couldn't help feeling affection for him. He was full of surprises. At the end of the interview, just before I left the office, when we were finishing with another topic altogether, he said again, "Hm! Boston! Heh-heh!" The interview had not been what I had expected.

After lunch a gaunt skeleton of a woman stumbled and fell into the ward between the arms of two male aides. "You come on now, up on your feet."

"I can't walk, please, call the doctor, get me some medicine," she said. "Give me a shot."

"Oh, Irene, you back here again? Shame on you, now!" one of the aides said, without looking up from her knitting.

Irene stopped writhing and said in a normal voice, "Hello,

Miss Kinney. I guess I just couldn't stay away." She twisted her hands together and laughed nervously.

"Well, I am disgusted with you. And look at you, you lost so much weight, you're skin and bones."

"I lost thirty pounds."

"But you wasn't fat, woman! What did you go and do that for?"

Irene flung out her arms and tried a delicate pirouette like a ballet dancer, as if half proud of her bony body, but stumbled before the turn was half done. She began to tremble all over. Her lips shook, her eyes filled with tears. She turned her profile like an actress sensing the location of a hidden camera. In her disarray she seemed to bring out different pieces of her personality to show us, like presents. Here is my grace, here is my pain, here is my beautiful face—but her face was no longer beautiful. Her eyes were huge, but the eyelids were thin and red, ringed with eyeliner in a ragged black line that traced the tremor of her hand as a graph on the tape of an electrocardiogram traces terminal heart disease. Her nose, once pert and slender, was knifelike. The nostrils were pinched and chapped. Orange dyed hair slipped over one eye and strands stuck against the red lipstick. The face paint pointed up the shape of her skull, which was ready to break through the tight skin over her forehead. She might have been a corpse tricked out for a wake by a drunken undertaker. From time to time she grabbed her narrow lower lip under her rabbit teeth.

Other patients had gathered in a circle to watch her. Ordinarily most patients ignored new arrivals (time enough to meet: they wouldn't be leaving soon), but Irene was different, she pulled our attention to her. She dropped her voice and affected a Southern accent. "I was so mis'ble, Miz Kinney. The day I left here, I went back on the pills."

"You looked so good when you left last time, you were just fine."

"I'm an addict. I'm an addict," Irene said very quietly. The moment passed: she shuddered, she doubled over and began to whine, "Get me some medication, nurse, please. I want paralde-hyde."

The sweet, heavy smell of the sedative was identifiable every-where Irene went. It summoned up images of funeral parlors in small towns, so precise was the odor. Alcoholics call paraldehyde an easy drunk, and are given it as they dry out here.

Miss Kinney said to herself, "That Irene, she always wants paraldehyde. That's for people who drink, not people who take pills. There's just no knowing about people's preferences." Irene staggered down the hall to her bed, supporting herself by cling-ing to the wall, and from time to time grabbing at the foot of a bed left out in the hallway. Mrs. Briggs, emerging from her room with tears in her eyes, watched the slow progress. "Wel-come to this hell," she said in a muddy voice.

Dr. Kegan was trying to work his way from the interview rooms to the big locked door like a quarterback maneuvering in a crowded field. While Irene cried for her medicine, I looked for a way out of mine. At the very least, four times a day, I wanted that option. I knew about Thorazine, I was finding out about loss of appetite compounding the miseries of hospital food, about lightheadedness and false euphoria, I could see other patients' skin as scaled as pale turtles' necks, and knew mine might be soon like theirs. This morning Luisa had been hopping down the hall with her tongue sticking out, a purple bladder swollen in front of her face, her breath wheezing around its perimeter as if the bulk of it came close to cutting off oxy-gen. Miss Kearnes had said, "Put your tongue back in your head!" in a rage at her insolence, but she had been stopped by Miss Kinney. "That's a drug reaction. Don't you know a Thora-zine overdose when you see one?" No, I didn't want to risk that; nor did I want to accept those rewards the drug gave us (who were properly dosed), of cotton-wrapped senses and naps that smothered; and yet, I could not commit myself to shunning the drug for the rest of my stay. Sooner or later I, the only one awake in a field of walking sleepers, would attempt murder. To be young, and strong, and physically caged, and to feel it

71

in my muscles, every minute, would turn me violent. And so I wanted to choose, each day, if I could stand it without the drug, or if I wanted to take it. When it was in liquid form, I had to swallow it. I grabbed at Dr. Kegan's coattails, a petitioner like the rest, and begged him to order my Thorazine given me as the little orange pills, "because the liquid is so bitter." He said yes, and it was done.

Purely as an experiment I asked for a pencil, an envelope, a piece of paper. I wrote to Helen. I wrote trivia about visiting hours, and the ward routine. I added a paragraph of information about other patients and staff members. I named names. If the hospital were to censor any letters at all, they must censor mine. I knew some prisons black out obscenity from inmates' mail, and I stopped short of planting such language only because it would seem out of character. There was no question in my mind: any curious person might wish to know who read her mail. I would ask Helen on the telephone just when my letter arrived, and if the envelope showed signs of having been unsealed. I licked the flap and pressed it shut with special care, and handed it to the nurse with the pencil.

A brief nap during visitors' hours got me through the disappointment of having no one come to see me. I knew, logically enough, that Helen could not come to visit often; a trip to Bellevue across town could take the best part of her working day. But foolish as the hope was, I kept listening for my name to be called out every time the elevator doors opened outside the locked door. By now it was hard to keep a real sense of an office workday in my mind; a ward routine seemed far more vivid.

I was awakened some moments before supper by a commotion in the hall. Mrs. Briggs was cringing in her dirty bathrobe in the midst of a circle of nurses and aides. Miss Sendell was saying, "You have to take your medication, Mrs. Briggs."

"I won't! I don't need that! I know what that is, it's Thorazine. You think I'm crazy, and I am *not* crazy. I won't take your Thorazine, I don't need it!"

Miss Sendell said with untroubled patience, "We've let you

refuse your pill for three days now, but the time has come. Either you take the medicine in pill form or we give you an injection."

"I want to talk to that doctor. I want to ask him if he thinks I'm a lunatic. You understand, don't you, that he's not fit to practice medicine. He prescribed Dilantin for me. Did he think I was an epileptic? Now he wants me to take Thorazine. Is he trying to poison me? He ought to have his license taken away. Let me talk to him. Let me tell him that!"

Miss Sendell conferred with some other nurses. Another nurse, who looked more official, joined the group. The circle of uniforms moved in a little closer. The supervisor said that she would listen to whatever Mrs. Briggs wished to say. Everyone was very calm except for Mrs. Briggs, whose voice rose and quivered. She looked so desperately for an escape route that her eyeballs rolled in her head.

"Which do you want, Mrs. Briggs, the pill or the injection?" asked Miss Sendell, with the large hypodermic ready in her hand.

"Nothing! Nothing! I'm not a lunatic!" screamed Mrs. Briggs. "Let me talk to my lawyer! I'll sue you!"

"This is perfectly legal, Mrs. Briggs. If necessary, we will put you in the jacket. For your own sake, I wish you'd accept this."

By now the nurses and aides were close enough to reach out their arms and hold Mrs. Briggs against the wall. One of the aides held a white canvas strait jacket. She didn't make a point of it, she kept it half behind her back, as if to spare Mrs. Briggs the sight of it. But Mrs. Briggs spotted it, her eyes were riveted on it, then flicked over to the hypodermic resting with its pad of cotton in the hand of the nurse. "Do you really think I'm a lunatic?" she asked, no longer defiant. "Am I a crazy person?"

"No, Mrs. Briggs, you aren't a crazy person, but you've had a rough time and you need some medication, that's all."

It was the calmness that got to her, finally, one could see that. That very calm people could produce strait jackets and hypodermics was enough to cause doubt. "Do you think I'm a lunatic?" she asked again, in a whisper. Then she took hold.

73

"All right," she said. "I will consent to the Thorazine, the pill. The hypodermic is highly objectionable. I will be in contact with my lawyer tomorrow, and with my private physician, and I will tell them precisely what has transpired this evening. Remove that hypodermic. You put this on the record, that I did take this of my own volition, but only under protest, under threat!" The nurses stood so still I heard the gulp in her throat as she washed down the pill with water from the paper cup. The staff moved away as quietly as they had gathered.

Mrs. Briggs, whom I had just watched in complete humiliation, recovered quickly. A moment ago she had almost believed she was insane. (I did not know, for fact, if she was, or if it mattered.) Now she was talking to the new addict, Irene Tompkins. Over and over she recited the tale, told of the doctor's stupidity, his barbarism, diagnosed her own case as one of understandable grief. "I hadn't been well, and last Thursday I received a telephone call. My dearest friend had been killed in an automobile accident. Of course I took some medication! But I wasn't trying to kill myself. Only a fool would try to commit suicide with an overdose of tranquilizers. I am not a fool. I didn't take Nembutal, I took meprobamate." Each time she reached one phrase—"I was just trying to blot out the pain"—the tears gushed from her eyes, her face collapsed in tears. Perhaps the Thorazine was taking effect, or perhaps by the fourth telling her story had worked on her like an incantation exorcizing her demon. Her chin shook, but her tone was reasonable. "I was just trying to blot out the pain." She was ready to hear a response; she had presented her case.

Irene said, "You have to do what they say if you want to get out of here, even if you know they're wrong. The medication probably won't hurt you, and they won't let you out unless you take it. You'll have to apologize to the doctor. You have to say, 'I apologize for my hostility,' or they won't let you out."

"But I'm not hostile!" said Mrs. Briggs, her voice running up the scale again.

"Well, they *think* you're hostile, so you have to work around that."

"I am not hostile. I am, considering these provocations, courteous. That fool, that dummkopf, is a dangerous man. He shouldn't be allowed possession of a license. I'm justified, I tell you!" Irene laughed at her, but gently. Mrs. Briggs stopped presenting her case. She put forth a compromise. "I'll say, 'I apologize for my hostile attitude, and don't think I'm saying that just so you'll let me out, because if you think that, you won't let me out and you'll defeat my whole purpose.'"

That was not quite a joke. Irene rehearsed her once again. "You say, 'I apologize for my hostile attitude,' and then stop." Mrs. Briggs learned her lines, laughing a little now and again, pretending she was playing a game, but simultaneously really learning the game, memorizing her part.

Doubtless Dr. Kegan based his diagnoses on factors quite other than rudeness, or apologies, but Irene believed that Mrs. Briggs was in Bellevue because she was stiff-necked, and there might be some truth to that: if she weren't arrogant and small-minded and stubborn, perhaps she would have married for love instead of money, there would have been children, perhaps she would have been comforted by her husband rather than an open-ended prescription of meprobamate. I had the feeling she had swallowed those pills to show she still could grieve; she'd prove it if it killed her. But even if Irene was wide of the mark, the simple truth was that Mrs. Briggs listened to her, and she was deaf to the doctor. If Irene wanted her to give up her will, she would remake herself if she could, because she trusted Irene, because Irene was a patient. Certainly after a session with Irene, Mrs. Briggs was easier to live with. Here there seemed no criteria for health or illness, the symptoms varied so, and opinions might differ. I thought health might be less a state of being than the process of becoming something other. Everything rigid, flat, inflexible that partook of death, and mirrored death, must be trampled like the enemy inhabiting the television set Mrs. Foster had attacked; surely Luisa, pulling the crisp white hair of the little old lady she was even now approaching again, arms outstretched, eyes blank, surely Luisa went to meet the same enemy; our life was regained not by drugging our bodies into a state of health but by working out new paths of action. Our lives might turn around no pattern but one of ragged and unfinished battle.

Mrs. Briggs tried again. "I can't succumb to the whims of that doctor."

"Well," Irene said, "you just have to figure out who's the right one to fight."

At dinner, Mrs. Briggs sat next to Irene and talked louder and more cheerfully than anyone else.

Could it be that there was some bond that tied us together, us patients, no matter our background or our values, something that made us more caring of one another? Certainly here Irene spent hours of patient talk with Mrs. Briggs, and even Mrs. Briggs, despite her complaints, was getting along. She heaved vocabulary around like cement blocks—let us never forget she was used to fancier company!—yet she passed the time of day with deaf, fat, depressed Mrs. Grumbacher with the beetle brows and the hearing aid, and unwittingly she was kind; if she was bored she hid it well. To see her attention focused on Harold, a droopy visitor from O 7, was to recognize how she would undertake a conversation with Bertrand Russell, but if you suggested this to her, she would deny it, just as I would bemoan my hours with Norma June discussing bubble gum, yet spend them just the same.

To amuse myself I took an informal poll. I asked patients if they felt more generous or tolerant here than in the outside world, and if they thought other people were more tolerant with them. I asked them if they ever felt like hitting another patient, or screaming at her. As I made my tour of the corridor, casually striking up conversations, I was glad for my patient's dress. I didn't hear what I expected, but I believed the answers were honest ones.

Everyone I talked to responded much the same way. Selina Jenks, the addict who had committed herself, interested me especially because she was not here for psychotic behavior, and because she was so blunt about hating it here. If anyone could see clearly the grimness of this ward, it would surely be she.

She said, "I want to get out of this dump. This place is full of shit. The patients—well, they're just a bunch of crazy people. They don't hurt nobody. No, you can't get mad with them, they do what they can. When they make *me* start to go crazy, I stop looking at them. They are all around, everywhere, but I get so I don't hear them."

Flo snuffled down the corridor like a rooting pig. Her bright little eyes glittered. "You got any food? Won't you give something to a hungry girl?"

Stupidity and malevolence rode behind those glittering eyes; surely some part of that dim brain kept score of the moods and nerves vibrating uneasily behind her retreating back. She demanded not food but our energy and our time. Here we were, some three dozen disparate ladies in a space twenty might find too small for comfort, no privacy, no space to hide, nothing familiar here from our daily lives, the people and the very food alien to us; we were depressing to look at, we were messy—because we were not allowed bobby pins or barrettes, our hair was tied back with string—we were depleted by tranquilizers and boredom, and afflicted with such a pitiful and morbid collection of tics, tremors, and meaningless cries, no one could blame us if we struck out with rage and impatience. How could we be expected to succor this gross animal who pulled at us like the meanest sort of plot against us: if the devil could not take us by direct assault, he would make Flo his instrument, and wear us down. So it seemed to me, and yet I could find no hostility toward her in my fellow patients.

Now she was heading for me, scratching at the pimples on her forehead. She whined, "I want to talk to you. Say something nice to me. I don't want to be alone." It was quite possible she was laughing at me. She might be saying to herself, "I have her now! How can she withstand a poor girl like me!" Thus she ate away at our reserves the way she ate away at the apples Helen brought me, or all of Norma June's Life Savers. It was all perfectly clear. And yet . . . and yet I did not turn her away. I talked to her about anything that came into my mind that might amuse her, I told her stories about places far from this ward. I told her things to amuse myself, about Paris at just this time of year, about the flowers in the gardens, and (knowing her interests) I talked about the food—the crêpes one could buy on street corners, dripping with sugar and rum, and strawberry tarts. I told her about walking over the bridge to the old markets before dawn, and seeing the sun rise blood-red over the stalls. I talked about one day when we would all be better, and we would live in happy homes. "Will I have a man? I want a man that will treat me good, and won't beat me up." I said I thought there was a good chance of that, we each might have a good man, and need never be hungry for anything again. "I'd like to live in those gardens, with the flowers," she said. All possibilities were equal to her, and equally unreal. It was like a fairy tale. She hadn't been out of New York City, except to travel to institutions in cars from other institutions.

"My name isn't Flo Tamis. I don't know why they call me that. I'm really Marie Rosten. When I was three years old, I was playing with my girl friend. She was four years old, and she was Jewish. We was up in the Projects, in the Bronx, you know where I mean? I lived up there in one of the buildings, but we got lost, we was playing in the lobby of one of the buildings. All the buildings looked so big, we never got found again. Somewhere there was a mother looking for her little Marie, and she never came home. They put me in a foster home and called me Flo Tamis. I don't know what happened to my girl friend. She was Jewish."

It probably wasn't true, but it might as well have been. Here I kept hearing stories that didn't square with facts, but one might prefer them to facts. No facts could pin down what was wrong with most of us, or what made us better, if we got better, and perhaps our true histories lay in our fantasies, along with the secrets of our disordered psyches. I couldn't rid my mind of the image of two small girls, running hand in hand around the corners of numberless giant buildings.

That night Miss Kearnes ordered us to bed again, right on time. Everyone fell asleep quickly; from the other room I could smell the odor of Irene's paraldehyde, sweet as ether. The creaking I had heard the night before picked up again, then stopped. I seemed to be the only one in the dormitory lying awake. Just before eleven I finally dozed off, but the smell of urine stung my nose again, and I recognized that this was no gift from a chronic bed-wetter in the bed beside me; this was stale, dried urine, weeks old. Beneath my head the mattress ticking was stiff as parchment. I leaped out of bed as if I had been scalded. Literally under my nose the whole time! Without bothering with my cardboard slippers I hurried down the corridor. Miss Kearnes was playing cards with Sally, Eileen, and Evelyn. I waited until they finished the bid.

"Miss Kearnes," I began.

"Wait a minute. Can't you see we're in the middle of this?"

I gathered insights into the criminal mind. I remembered how briskly we had been shooed to bed like children—except for the "well" patients who would amuse themselves with a hand of bridge. Oh, Miss Kearnes! You bully! Thick-faced, dull-witted, I'd sooner take Flo for my keeper. And the three girls, what traitors! Thieves! Playing cards with the jailer! "Three hearts," said Sally, as if I weren't there, she, too, in league to make me invisible. No, these three were not patients, they were some treacherous offspring to staff, well people pretending to be sick, perhaps, to spy on me! Was it so bizarre to imagine that I might be proved in fact unbalanced, while I waited meekly plotting murder, and these three girls, old hands at being sick, now showed up as well; they knew how to ease a path around Miss Kearnes, who ranked us with all the corruption of the law on the ward. I swore I'd sooner be locked in seclusion than play that game.

Yet still I waited. I wished I had put on my slippers. All my plots dissolved in self-pity and envy, and when the moment came, I gave in. I told lies, I smiled. "What do you want?" Miss Kearnes finally asked. She didn't look up from her cards. Phoebe had said about her, "She's okay, after you get to know her." But why should I have to get to know an aide before she would treat me like a human being?

"My mattress stinks of stale pee," I said. My tone was so

rude I covered it with a sweet smile. I was cousin to Uriah Heep.

"Well, what do you want me to do about it? I'm not going to scrub it down for you, that's for sure."

"I was looking for an extra sheet to cover it up with. The sheet I've got is too short, and I'm lying right on the mattress."

"Just let me finish this trick." Ten minutes later Miss Kearnes led me into the linen closet. Generously, she gave me a blanket as well. "Use this for a pillow, why don't you. That will get your face out of it. Wrap the sheet around it like a pillowcase, and you should do all right. Tomorrow, why don't you try turning the mattress?" Surely she was a pleasant enough person, as long as I was reasonable with her; but as I was deciding that Phoebe was right, that she was okay when you got to know her, I remembered that we had lost our reason, we were here because we were not reasonable. So I said good night, thanked her too many times, and went back to bed.

Five

In my mind I had framed angry speeches until close to three in the morning. I reacted too strongly to everything here. I cared too much about the people I trusted—Luisa, Jeannette, Priscilla (was it chance that drew me closest to schizophrenia?)—and I was periodically suspicious of even the kindest staff member. I ran through scenarios of being exposed as a fraud, and taken off to jail. I lived in a state of high melodrama. The more desperate I grew for decent civilized conversation, the more I needed to share what was in my mind, the less able I seemed to reach out to those staff members who seemed to want to like me. Worn out by thinking about these matters, I slept through the bell again, through the shouts of the aides, and Evelyn shook me so hard I almost fell out of bed.

In the bathroom, Priscilla was once again sitting on the floor by the toilets. She giggled at some inner joke, and seemed cheerful. When I approached her, she looked as if I had interrupted her. Leola Gibson washed her face, wiped it on the sheet the aide held up, and tried to get Priscilla to do the same. "Come here, child, and get ready for your breakfast."

Priscilla frowned. "Go 'way, le' me 'lone, 'm busy. Busy." It was the closest thing to English that she had spoken since I'd been in the hospital. I could believe she was busy. As I watched her face, she was holding a dialogue with herself about something important, and learning things from one part of her nature that amused another part. Perhaps it had been the latest visit from her mother that set her off. Mrs. Pyle had confronted the doctor; there had been a scene. The doctor had advised a state hospital, and Mrs. Pyle swore she would fight it. She wore a cloth coat, much too long, very worn, but she had an intense, intelligent face and thin nervous lips. After she left, the aides grumbled about her. "That woman is all trouble. You can see where Priscilla's troubles come from." Perhaps Priscilla's new mood was bound up with some new thing she had learned these past few days about her mother and herself, and what they knew that the world didn't.

I liked Priscilla, perhaps because few others did. The other ladies did not find her good company because she was "busy," because she didn't invite or accept ordinary conversation, and because she spent most of her time borrowing cigarettes and asking for lights. Sometimes she stole cigarettes from people's belongings, or was suspected of it. Only Norma June took pains with her. Norma June would instruct her on the proper way to brush her teeth, would try to get her hair combed, and sometimes, when Priscilla allowed it, put lipstick on her. It was difficult to tell if Priscilla appreciated what Norma June told her, but since she was docile enough, she might have been grateful for the kind intention.

"You get going, now, Priscilla, wash your face good. I'm going to be leaving today, maybe, or tomorrow, and I want you to look good."

Leola, oblivious to symptoms, asked, "You going home, sister?"

"I'm being transferred to University Hospital," said Norma June. "I like it here all right, but my husband thinks I'll do better there, I don't know why. I'm sure trying here. I'm trying just as hard as I can to get better. I didn't give anything away last night, and I wanted to so bad." My standards had shifted so since I had come here that a private hospital seemed unconscionable luxury. Mr. Jacobsen must have loved Norma June as much as she said he did, to spend that money. He was a contractor, but times were hard, and he hadn't been getting the work he needed. "He's my third husband," Norma June told me. "It's like I never was married before. I feel like somebody on the *Newlywed Game* with him, and we've been married seven years. I sure am lucky. He'd do anything for me. I just hope I can go home to him soon, because he misses me so much."

At breakfast, Leola Gibson rapped on the table with her big spoon. Conversation died down. "Everybody be quiet, because I'm going to say grace this morning." Some people put down their spoons. Luisa and Jeannette Rosetti bowed their heads and folded their hands. They closed their eyes. "Blessed Lord, please, now, you look out after all these sisters here, and bless them, and in your infinite mercy guide their steps. Bless this food that we have to eat, and praise be it's here for us to eat, and it is pretty fine food, even if it isn't as good as what we gets for ourselves at home. Amen." Several patients said amen politely. Spoons were raised once again over oatmeal and cold scrambled eggs.

After a pause, Leola began again. "Sisters, the Lord, speaking through my mouth, says everyone is to put three butters and three salts on their oatmeal this morning." Phoebe laughed out loud. Several other ladies covered their smiles with their napkins.

Norma June thought it over before she said, dead serious, "Gibson, I think that's going a little too far."

Several other people laughed and Leola looked confused. "Well, maybe you're right. That's too much." She reconsidered.

"You only have to put one butter and one salt on your oatmeal this morning, sisters."

After the morning shower I was handed a dress even longer than the one the day before. I tended to trip over the hem. My friend the student nurse suggested I hem it in occupational therapy, and pointed out a room in the corridor between the male and female sides of the floor. Here was where Gerta had made her bag.

The room was jammed with shabby equipment, supplies for crafts, and patients. There was a 1922 Underwood typewriter on a table, a pegboard covered with samples of patients' leatherwork, an ancient Singer sewing machine, a table covered with construction paper, pots of glue, pieces of string. A tall cabinet was stuffed with scraps of material and balls of yarn. Around the walls were drawings and watercolors, sewn samplers, plaques of clay painted with watercolors. The room was tiny, but held perhaps a dozen patients, men as well as ladies. Eddie, my friend from the first day on the ward, was sewing a vinyl wallet with a plastic thong made to look like leather. Miss Pickman was the occupational therapist in charge, a cool handsome young woman who said, "You can't cut off that dress unless you get permission from a nurse." Miss McMullen looked flustered. A student nurse obviously didn't count as a nurse. I veered off on a half-hour search for a nurse willing to give me permission to cut six inches off my dress. Finally one said, "It's a silly idea, but I won't stop you." I was allowed to use the scissors under Miss Pickman's eye, but I must do all the sewing in the occupational therapy room. I was not allowed to take a needle into the ward. I was caught between my sweet student nurse on one side, who sat down beside me to help me along with comforting conversation, whether I wished it or not, and my friend Eddie on the other.

Eddie said, "Why don't you make a wallet like this? Or you can make a pocketbook or a dress." Eagerly he showed me each artifact in turn. He is trying to take me over, I thought stubbornly. He has to tell people what to do. He has to show people he knows a better way.

A big black man with a scar on his cheek said, "Leave her alone, Eddie. She don't want to make a pocketbook. Let people be."

Doing a job of work was almost overwhelming; a task, with a beginning, a middle, an end, and then a result to live with. A responsibility. My hands were shaking while I used the scissors. I tried to conceal it by working quickly. To my horror, when I made the circuit and held up the gown against my body, it was too short, it was the length of a pajama top. Like a nightmare a childhood pattern of reactions took me over. Panic, the threat of tears, the urge to run away. The consequences were unthinkable! I would be punished in some way, someone would scold me. I would be held up as an example. I would never be allowed in the occupational therapy room again. Everyone would see me wearing my bathrobe tied shut through the day instead of my nightgown, and would ask me why. I would have to confess to destroying hospital property.

The man with the scar was watching me. "Well now, I think that's just about the right length," he drawled. "I'd like to see you try that on." I almost hugged him for his good humor. I made myself take hold. "You're crazy, Anne," I told myself. "You're acting like a little child. What is the worst that can happen to you? The worst already *has* happened to you, you're here in Bellevue, and you're doing fine. There's nothing more you have to be afraid of."

"I think this gown needs a ruffle," I said to Miss McMullen, as we both eyed the dress judiciously. I trimmed several inches from the piece lying on the floor, leaving the machine hem intact. When I tacked the strip back on the dress, it was exactly the right length.

The man looked disappointed. "I liked it better the other way. I thought you was going to give old Sam a look at your pretty legs."

Sam Buck watched me sew. He asked, "Now what are you doing?"

It seemed plain enough to me, so I said, "I'm mending a strait jacket." The man laughed and Miss McMullen looked concerned.

85

"You fixing that for me?" Sam said.

"I'm afraid it's a lady's model, but I'll work on one for you if you give me a day or two."

"Naw, I want one with pretty flowers. Maybe we can share that one. Let me get inside that one with you." He gave me a look both lascivious and merry, and it was my turn to laugh.

"Now I know why I've got a chaperone," I said, nodding at Miss McMullen, who gave in and laughed, too. For the first time in days—it seemed weeks—I felt female, warm, and attractive. I had every confidence that the man did not see the hospital pallor in my skin or my chapped white lips, just as I noticed his twinkling eyes, and overlooked the wrinkled blue pajamas knotted at the waist (the buttons were long since lost) and the nappy untended hair. He looked handsome enough for me, and because his skin was black, he escaped the unhealthy pallor I shared with Eddie and the other white patients. He was at home in this institution. I guessed he'd been in prisons, it was an intuition, and I wondered where he'd come from, to ride so well on this routine.

At last the hem was finished. I felt like Penelope, the skirt was so voluminous. Miss McMullen stole a look at her watch, and I wanted to tell her she didn't have to sit with me, but she felt it her duty, and she did it. I left Sam teaching Eddie how to play chess. He offered to teach me some other day. He said he'd learned the game when he was in San Quentin, so I knew he'd made the big time.

Back on the ward, Norma June berated Miss Hargins. "There's shit all over the bathroom. Somebody got shit all down the side of the toilet, and didn't clean it up."

Phoebe called out, "Baby Snooks did it," pointing at Miss Hargins.

Evelyn started to giggle. "Baby Snooks! Baby Snooks! That's a good name for you!"

Miss Hargins looked craven. "I didn't do nothing, I didn't do nothing, I was just standing here, I don't know what you're talking about," she babbled in a little baby voice. Her sandy eyebrows shot up on her forehead. "What are you looking at me for?"

"You're just too nasty," Norma June said. "Don't let her have a cigarette," she said peremptorily to Jeannette Rosetti, who was always ready to be used. "She can't have a cigarette until she cleans up that mess. She has diarrhea because she don't eat good, and because she won't listen to nobody. Why, she can't even tell you her own name." Miss Hargins mumbled gently to herself. Norma June was growing more frantic as time passed. Here she was, leaving the ward so soon, and there were so many tasks undone! So many failings to correct and frail spirits to support! "Don't let anybody light that cigarette she's carrying around because she stole it. She took it from Earthalee's pocketbook, and I watched her do it. Now she don't remember her name, so we're going to give her a new one."

Leola Gibson suggested we call her Cindy. Norma June said, "Okay, we're going to call you Cindy. But not until you clean up that shit, and wash your hands nice, and come out here and sit down. If you don't do it right, we won't call you Cindy, we'll call you Nasty."

The task of reforming Miss Hargins seemed quixotic, particularly as some of the ladies didn't like Norma June much more than they liked Miss Hargins. Nonetheless, Norma June instantly had organized the group into an effective boycott. No one lit Miss Hargins' cigarette, no one moved over to let her sit down on the orange chairs, no one spoke to her. Luisa, hopping down the hall on one foot, was the only one too busy with her own affairs to pay attention. Miss Hargins seemed unaware of her disgrace. She was hallucinating again. She babbled, and shook her skinny fist in the air. "Why didn't you listen to me, like a good boy!" she said. It looked like a lost cause.

"Stop talking like that, Nasty," Norma June said. "Go clean up that shit."

Miss Hargins cocked her head slyly and said, "I'm going to speak to the Governor about you." And shuffled off down the hall. But when she was almost past the bathroom, she hesitated, looked around like a thief, and slipped inside. We heard a great clattering and the sound of water running. I passed by the bathroom and saw the old lady daubing at the wall and the floor behind the toilet. She muttered and quarreled with the feces on the sponge. Norma June waited with arms akimbo until Miss Hargins doddered back down the hall, stopping as if by accident in front of Norma June to repeat her threat about the Governor.

Norma June said, "You didn't wash your hands, and you left some shit on the side of the toilet. You did a little, so we won't call you Nasty, but we won't call you Cindy, either." Now that was a fair and serious judgment. I imagined that had the decision been up to me, I might have praised the old lady for honest effort, and hated her secretly for her meanness, and for the mean sweet smell of diarrhea that clung about her person.

In the morning I telephoned my minister and told him where I was. The wall telephone had been repaired at last, and those who had dimes could call whenever they wished. He told me that he would come to see me. Aside from the fact that we were friends, he was a good visitor to have, for his clerical collar would gain him admittance at any time. Ministers and priests don't have to wait for visiting hours. My new life was so circumscribed that it seemed a miracle that someone could come in and out without asking permission. I asked him to bring me a book with wide margins, because I wished to take some notes. (My copy of *The Idiot* was a cheap paperback crammed with type, and I had used up the flyleaves and the inside of the covers.) I asked him to make it something dull about religion, to discourage people from prying into it, and he agreed, and it wasn't until I hung up the telephone that I realized this was not tactful to say to a minister.

Before lunch I went into the dormitory. Maxine was crawling out of the next bed to go to work. Maxine was different from the rest of us, for she had a pass to go out to work as a barmaid each afternoon. As a consequence, I had seen her rarely, and didn't know her at all. She was nineteen, and already half her attention was on the outside world. Each day she slept through breakfast undisturbed by aides. Each noon she awakened, stretched like a cat, and put on her clothes, layer by layer, in a ritual that never varied. It was a religious rite. First underwear, slimpsy lace in red or black from the dime store, or from one of those shops on Forty-second Street that specialize in bikini underpants and bras with peekaboo openings for the nipples. A dress of cotton or thin synthetic material that she had made in occupational therapy. Threads hung off the uneven hem, and the side seams were sewn up by hand. The dress had no shape of its own, but clung at the bust and hips, and was very short. The make-up went on, layer by layer, until the fresh skin was stopped up with beige base, the pores plugged with powder, and the natural blush buried underneath was painted fresh on top of everything, a feverish burn along the cheekbones. The black eyebrows were plucked out one by one, and in their place a black pencil line, highly arched. Three shades of eye shadow, false eyelashes top and bottom, and black eyeliner turned large bright eyes into caverns. Last there was the hair, and this varied every day. Sometimes it was combed long over the cheeks, sometimes snarled into a two-foot beehive. Usually a spit curl was stuck on cheek or forehead with Scotch tape. A generous dash of perfume that smelled like musk, and Maxine could face the world. The mouth never smiled; it was frozen in a pout by Pink Passion lipstick and Frosted Gloss that she applied in three layers.

This attention to the details of dress was so rare on the ward that patients often stood in a silent ring around Maxine to watch. Today a patient she disliked started a conversation. Maxine ignored her. Her sullenness was a defensive weapon that we all used often. We did not insult or berate one another, but we might answer a question with a blank expression. It was a way to keep peace, and to keep our privacy. Most of us turned our thoughts inward, and talked much less than on the outside; many of us were quarreling with our own demons, or hiding from them by sinking into apathy. I did it, too: I would sit in one spot and stare into space from time to time, just as I did the first day in the hospital, willing myself numb. It was a rest from frustration and paranoia. It was the easiest way to keep individual privacy. Sometimes we all needed to talk, to say some crazy thing, or just to say hello to another person. Sometimes we needed to be alone with our thoughts. Each of us developed an uncanny sense of another's mood, and a feeling for the ability of others to respond. Maxine liked to talk to Evelyn and Phoebe, and her best friend was Eileen Thibeau. They would lie on Maxine's unmade bed and talk about their pasts and their troubles.

At noon Jeannette Rosetti was calm and lucid after her medication. She walked up to join the circle of ladies watching Maxine put on her make-up. Because she was pretty, the ladies liked to look at her. Sometimes they came closer, stared, measured the psychic distance between them, and backed off, saying nothing. Jeannette Rosetti said, "I was really sick yesterday."

Maxine added a bow on the top of her beehive. She didn't answer. Jeannette picked up no animosity. The silence said, "I hear you, and I'm not very interested. I'll put up with you, though, if you don't care if I ignore you."

Jeannette said, "Gee, I thought I was Jesus's wife. I thought my boy friend was Gabriel. I guess I know something now, I know I'm pretty fucked up."

Maxine turned her back. Jeannette walked down the hall without bitterness. A moment later Maxine said to no one in particular, "I don't know why they all come up to me." She was still facing the wall.

I was finishing my dessert at lunch with the rest of the ladies and I knew I had a visitor because quiet little Mrs. Feeny, the brunt of Luisa's physical attacks, called out, "Father! Father! Bless me, Father!" in a reedy little voice, and there in the doorway I saw Michael Allen. Although he wore a surplice for church services, he almost never wore a clerical collar, and he looked slightly uncomfortable in it today, and uncomfortable with his surroundings. For an instant I saw us all through his eyes, grey ghosts, staring at him, calling out to him, trying to leach out of him the particular blessing that collar promised, and he, frail enough vessel himself, was doubtless working to remember that these were God's children, too, although they looked like creatures of the devil, swatting at imaginary flies, slopping their soup, hiding bits of bread under their dresses, or talking nonsense to the air. As my friend, he had been put on the spot.

We sat at a corner table in the dining room and carved out some privacy by talking very quietly. I was oppressively conscious of Jeannette Rosetti, Luisa, and Leola waiting politely across the room for a chance to speak to Father Allen. For a moment we found some peace. He handed me a paper bag that contained some apples and a paperback entitled *Man's Need and God's Action,* by Reuel L. Howe. It had a blank page at each chapter opening.

Michael was under a dual pressure. For any outsider, the sight of us! I responded to his reaction by trying to explain (No, it's not the way it looks—the ladies are very nice, I have friends here), and whatever I said seemed as vacuous as a patient's stare, and did not explain anything at all. We patients tended to be inarticulate.

But Michael was under the tension also of knowing why I was in this place, and how I got here. He had to quell his doubts about the legitimacy of the project while at the same time offering me his version of pastoral comfort. I had asked him to walk into my research project as he walked into the ward and figure out on short notice many of the questions I had been thinking about for weeks. I felt I had been unfair to ask this of him.

We talked about activities at the church, and Michael, noticing my paperback of *The Idiot,* told me about a time when that book was important to him, when he was working in a psychiatric hospital. We talked about ideas. My uneasiness with him fell away. It seemed weeks since my brain had worked quite this hard in quite this way, and it was a wonderful feeling. I needed this; without people like Michael, or the books I couldn't read here, part of my brain would atrophy. I knew it, and I wondered how people lived for months and years in institutions and emerged able to think. Prisoners I had known had spent hours in prison libraries, but I doubted that I, had I been forced to spend months here, would have had the will to read in these overcrowded quarters.

Being in some ways a modest man, Michael wouldn't have chosen to spend the last fifteen minutes of his time on N 7 blessing patients, but one by one they lined up, hands folded, head bowed, and it would have been cruelty to explain he was Episcopalian rather than Catholic. "Father, Father!" the cry went up, like the mewing of cats, and he put out a hand and blessed each petitioner. At the locked door I thanked him again for coming, and he said he'd come again. "You know, if you don't have anything else to do, you might read the Howe. It's actually not a bad book," he added wistfully.

In the early afternoon Norma June made herself ready for the transfer to University Hospital. Her anxiety had been mounting throughout the day. Mattie Jackson helped her by scrubbing down the fixtures in the bathroom. Mrs. Jackson approached the task with the pride of a professional. She started with the scratched metal mirrors, polishing them with a sheet, and worked her way down the wall to the spigots, the basin. It was difficult to remove the stains with Ivory soap, but that was all she was allowed, and she was methodical and scrubbed for a long time.

Mrs. Foster had spent one night in seclusion, and was now being given another chance on the ward. She was certainly logical today. She said, "Mattie, you're a damn fool to do all that work. In ten minutes, somebody going to stop up the drain or shit in it, you know that. I wouldn't do that dirty work for nobody!" But Mrs. Jackson had her pride. No militant she, but the finest lady's maid, ordering her life around service and a starched uniform, cleanliness and common sense. So she must see herself, as she faced down Mrs. Foster's mocking voice. Her small round face was serious and prideful. She had breeding. Mrs. Foster lived by energy picked up from the street, but Mrs. Jackson had learned her style in a white lady's kitchen. Or so said the set of her chin and the straightness of her back.

"I like to keep a clean place," she said. The words were not distinct. A cleft palate blurred the words, and left its mark on her scarred upper lip, drawn up to one side and swollen as if she had been struck there. Her nose was flattened down to meet it slightly off center above the seam, and attached to it by a thin whitened line. Mrs. Jackson was tough, all right, but she knew how to hide it, she knew how to act nice with white folks, and keep her place when she thought it to her advantage. Behind that honest, humble face lay hoarded wiles and plots.

Mrs. Foster gave an amiable grin. "Fuck," she said. "Ain't nobody here gonna pay no mind *what* you do."

"Well, she wanted it," Mrs. Jackson said with a nod toward Norma June, who was organizing a crew to mop up the water spilled from the drinking fountain. "She's going off to another hospital, and she wanted things to look good before she left."

Mrs. Foster hooted, then grinned again, a sly grin of complicity that Mrs. Jackson returned. "She sure do push," Mrs. Foster said.

"She'll push, and I'll give way," said Mrs. Jackson.

"Well, we know where she's at. Fuckin' old bitch, she can't help herself. She's going, anyway."

Like a whirlwind, Norma June inspected. Gaunt, stalking like a crane, she squinted at the sinks. "Now that looks real nice. You're real good at cleaning, not like some I could name who mess in their pants. From now on, Gerta, you do the inspecting, and Mrs. Jackson, you keep up with it. I won't be able to keep an eye on you all any more, but I know you'll be okay. You're going to get better real fast, I just know it. You keep on trying to help the nurses and the doctors, and don't give the aides no trouble, and you'll be out of here real soon." I wondered if Norma June was reading off in her mind what she hoped someone would say to her. The tension knotted chords in her thin neck. She wrung her hands as if she was afraid to let them free. She spoke to every patient, kissed most of us on the cheek, and gave out hugs. She took special pains to find me. "You all take care of this little girl, you hear? She's real sweet, and just you don't forget she's got no family. I want you all to be family to her." She hugged some of the aides, one of whom made a face behind her bony back.

"Sister, you look out for yourself, now," Leola Gibson sang out. "The Lord Jesus done told me you gonna do all right. You gonna get better real fast, because you gonna take your medication and do just what the doctor say. He told me that this morning."

Norma June said, "Gibson, I appreciate the sentiment. I hope sometime you stop spending so much time talking to Jesus, but if He helps you get better, you take His advice, as long as you're listening anyway."

"Thank you, sister, I know you always understand, and that's why the good Lord is blessing you today, even though you is a little hard to take sometimes. You're a little nervous, did you know that? You got to learn to take life easy."

Mr. Jacobsen arrived at last. He was tall and thin, built just like his wife, and every time he looked at her his face lit up with pride and love. After they left, the tension in the ward dissolved. There wasn't much conversation; apathy covered the ward like a blanket. I had grown so used to the drone of Norma June's voice I had stopped noticing it, but now that it was gone, the air shifted uneasily, small sounds became more noticeable, the shuffle of feet, the clatter of dishes in the pantry, all muffled by closed doors, a drowsy, half-expectant hush, like the mood in a room when a clock suddenly stops ticking.

The afternoon glided by. Visiting hours came and went. At 4:00 a social worker called me in to talk. It was not Miss Garber, but another girl, also young, pretty, and earnest. She didn't smile at all. She told me that Dr. Kegan would like to see my friend Helen, and I asked her about my prospects for getting out of the hospital soon. She said, "Of course, you understand that only the doctor is qualified to tell you that, Miss Barry." When I asked her to make a generalization of what the average stay was, she said that one could not make a rule, that each case was different. But perhaps she could tell me from her experience the shortest stay she could remember, if a patient had been discharged, say, within a week of admission. She hedged, she could not say. Many patients must badger her thus, and she knew better than to risk an opinion. What hopes she might arouse, what despair! But beyond the practical difficulties lay the simple truth that each patient was sick with a different disease, which the doctor himself could diagnose only in the most general terms, and although he might treat what he did not understand, he could not predict a result that he could not foresee. In my mind I fought this logic. Not I, I'm different, I am not really a patient, I am understandable, and if you give me a hint of what to do to appear better, I alone of your patients can do it. So ran the protest in my mind. And I could not say that without giving myself away, nor recognize an echo here of Mrs. Briggs' hysteria. My muscles grew tense with frustration. Would no one ever see that I was I, not like the others? I fought irritation with Miss Roy, and it took all my energy and attention to stay calm. I made my face blank and stupid, like a wall. Miss Roy said, "I can tell you that the doctor will probably want to see you again to see how you feel, but I don't know when that will be. I wouldn't plan on anything sooner than the end of next week, but that's not certain, of course, one way or another." The end of next week! I thought I had puzzled out every possibility, but here, apparently, logic never applied. Every decision was arbitrary. But it was impossible! I couldn't spend two weeks here! I could have cried.

Abruptly enough I was taken out of these unhappy thoughts by Mrs. Foster, who had once again been giving the staff trouble. Without her wig and her teeth, she lay strapped to a bed in the corridor. She asked me my name, and I told her. I knew her in her quiet moments as Mrs. Foster, but when she was violent she was a different person. I wanted to know if she saw herself that way, as two people in one skin, and if one personality knew the other, so I asked her name.

"I don't know," she said, "but whatever it is, it's Mister."

I prompted, "Mister Foster?"

"Just you call me Mister." She winked one eye half shut and said, "I'm going to kiss your sweet breast. And then I'm going to come all over my body."

For ten seconds I stood riveted with surprise—did I hear right? Then her face broke out in a grin, she chuckled down in her throat, let it grow, rolled the sound out in a self-satisfied rumble, like a tribute to the happiest sexual acts, a bawdy laugh, with some of the same mood I had heard in Sam Buck's voice this morning. I burst out laughing, too.

"You're just as bad as you can be, Mister Foster. If you let the nurse hear you talk like that, you'll get in all kinds of trouble."

"Oh, darling, I'm always in trouble. I thrives on trouble. I don't pay it no mind. In this place, I've got to have my fun."

Beyond missing Helen, I had felt the loneliness of having no one else to look forward to. I have in real life been spoiled by a fond family, and have as many friends as I might wish; under other circumstances I imagine I might have called ten, fifteen, two dozen people if I had wanted to, each willing to come to see me, try to get me transferred to a private hospital, signed out by a private psychiatrist; I hadn't known before how privileged a segment of society I moved in. I took it for granted. But now I noticed women with no visitors at all, and some with a husband or a daughter, but no friends eager to help, and even Mrs. Briggs, despite many hysterical calls to her mother, who presumably lived comfortably on the Upper East Side, was not being transferred to a private hospital. Of course I had told no one besides Michael and Helen of my plan, and so for once I shared only the small comforts of most of the patients here. But the conversation with Michael had cheered me, and I was able to compliment Jeannette Rosetti on her visitor with honest pleasure for her, and no envy at all.

"I liked the way he looked," I said. He had worn tight jeans, an army shirt torn in the sleeve, a leather vest with fringes hanging six inches below his belt, three chains of tiny glass beads about his neck, and a beaded band around his forehead. His hair was heavy and black, cut like an American Indian's, chopped off in bangs over his low forehead, and the rest hanging to his shoulders. He might have passed for a stocky Sioux. But when he spoke it was in Spanish—he was Puerto Rican, his usual haunt Gem's Spa, headquarters of hippieland on the Lower East Side, at Second Avenue and St. Mark's Place. On the ward he looked colorful and cocky, and I was grateful for his presence. Amid the drabness of the surroundings he stood out like a banner. He hid secrets in his heavy-lidded eyes, and when he smiled he seemed to be promising special treats to us patients. Some of the relatives who visited were afraid of us, or compassionate, almost all were nervous with any but their own sister or mother, as if that one patient were someone, a real person here by mistake amid a crowd of potentially dangerous animals. Most visitors hurried through the door and into the dining room without letting other patients catch their eye. I always said hello to Jeannette's boy friend and he always smiled that enigmatic smile at me. (What looked like nobility on the ward was brutality when I passed him on the street six months later. The heavy expression, the slow amble marked nothing more than hours and years spent with Thunderbird concealed in a brown paper bag. His clothes at that later time were spattered with mud, his jaw slack, his face brutalized by generations of bad blood and corruption, or so it seemed. In his wrecked brain the life force pulsed feebly, and charity had long since died, but in Bellevue I saw none of this. I took in his stumbling walk, his murmured greeting, and loved him like a brother.)

And so I was sincere when I told Jeannette about my feelings. "Thank you," she said, polite and close to Victorian in her charm. "He's my husband. He's my common-law husband. That's it." She laughed as if that were a joke. "I was playing my guitar on St. Mark's Place, on the sidewalk there, by the Spa. The rain was coming down. I remember the rain. I was playing for money. Sometimes I would go there and play, and people would give me nickels and quarters. He walked up to me and I never saw him before. He kissed me on the mouth and the rain kept coming down, it kept raining. I said, 'Maybe you'll be my man,' and he said yes. He didn't say yes, because he doesn't speak English, but he went home with me, and he stayed with me. He has a problem, with drinking. He was drunk when he kissed me, but then he was always drunk. He stopped last week, for me. He didn't use to know what he was doing. He's my husband, my common-law husband."

"How long have you been with him?" I asked her.

"Three months. I call him Cochise, because I think he looks like an Indian, but I don't know what other people call him. He doesn't speak English too good, so I never found out." The Thorazine was working on her; she was gentle and vague in her mood, but her sentences followed a line of thought. In an hour or so she would begin to drift away. The sentences would become fragments, the smile would flicker on and off like a light around her mouth, and her staring eyes would focus in midair as if she were watching a film.

I felt the greatest affection for Jeannette. She had no malice. Alone, of all the patients, she was always trying to figure out what was expected of her, and to do it. Her personality was clear as water, she was all love. During the bad times, she spoke of some of the things she saw. She offered up her mind like a bunch of flowers, Cassandra shuffling up and down the corridor. "He's coming," she'd say cheerfully, "Jesus is coming, and Gabriel. The time is at hand. You walk a long way. I listened to the music and God sang about it. Joseph is going to be there, and I'll be with them. I think it's time to go to Mass, if the candles are ready."

With the evening came a diversion. One of the aides brought in a portable record player that we set up in the hall between the men's and women's sides of the floor. The only furniture in that area was two battered wooden benches and a card table. Some people listened, others danced—the frug, the bugaloo, the funky Broadway. The music was black or Puerto Rican, it was soul music. Now that we no longer had the nattering of the television set hours each day, we could have this music. Otis Redding, B. B. King, Aretha Franklin, José Feliciano. Blues, the big sound of hard rock. Several of the ladies came shuffling out to listen, including some I would not have expected to see.

Belle Grumbacher, the large beetle-browed Jewish matron, turned up her hearing aid. Mrs. Feeny squeezed into a corner of the bench, pulling at her skirts so she wouldn't have to touch anyone, but she stayed even when Flo flopped down beside her. As whites, we were in the minority here. Evelyn and Sam danced, snapping their fingers. Evelyn worked in a modified bump and grind, a bit of the jerk, a bar or two of pure Harlem invention. No wonder we whites gathered to watch: there was an electricity in the air, funky sex and humor in the dancing, a beat to the music that set the dancers apart from us wasted onlookers. This is a black world with life we lost generations ago, if we ever had it. We sensed it, we reacted to it, we whose souls were in jeopardy, and we listened hoping that we could catch hold of that spirit and help ourselves. Ellis did his own dance, all by himself, camp ballet, but elegant and rich as silk. His coppery skin gleamed, the sweat rolled down his neck as he tucked in his chin and strutted like a rooster, spun on one toe, swooped, dipped, sashayed right and left. Sam said, "Come on, Big Mama," and swept an aide onto the floor. She laughed and pushed him away, but caught in the music like a leaf in the wind, she danced, too, shaking her wide hips and stomping. When Ellis bowed to Phoebe, and she leaned into a loose-jointed frug, other white people started to dance. As if on signal, we were admitted into the black world, a little reprieve for us, and I had the poignant memory of other days, before the civil rights movement failed. Before we traded in our black friends for racial guilt, we went to parties in Harlem with just this feeling. Eddie, who had pursued me the first day, asked me to dance, and so we did; several of the other aides joined in, and Flo Tamis did her own slouching steps, her big breasts rolling under her nightdress, and all the while she hummed off key to a Marva Whitney record called "It's My Thing (You Can't Tell Me Who To Sock It To)." Each in the shape of her own disease, restrained, depressed, manic, did her dance. We were allowed to stay up late, because the aides were enjoying the dancing as much as the patients. It was the first time I had felt so free in days.

Sometime in the middle of the night I woke up with a start to the sound of wild laughter. I froze in my bed, sure that some patient was roaming the wards, and would shortly be flung into isolation by the aides. But instead of the expected clatter and confusion, only the laughter rang out again, louder, and again. Another voice joined in. Stray words, the drone of several voices, some giggles. It was impossible to sleep. I crept out of bed and tiptoed out into the hall. The big clock said two-thirty. The sounds were nearer. They came from the social workers' office, and through the open door I saw the aides playing cards and talking. This was the night shift, who came on at midnight and left at eight in the morning. Because I now slept through until Evelyn woke me each day, I had not seen their faces before this moment; now they loomed up against the bright light from the desk shining over their cards. Each woman was huge; never had I seen such a collection of formidably large women, solid muscle under the fat, their shoulders stretching the blue uniforms, their skirts pulled tight over spread thighs as they leaned back in their seats (an ominous cracking at the shift of weight) and laughed at one aide's blunders in the game. I was present at a secret cabal, for indeed no patient should be afoot at two-thirty in the morning, there were rules against that, and a transgressor must be a spy to think of it, or mad, and there were ways to deal with the mad. But I was transfixed, catching the winking of light off eyeglass lenses, or off a gold tooth in a wide mouth flung back in a guffaw. "Shee-it, you don't know *nothing* about this game, you got us in a fix for sure!" One of the aides tipped her chair back on its rear legs to reach a transistor radio, turned the knob as far as it could go to pick up "Light My Fire," and hummed along with it.

Swiveling back to the game, she spotted me standing in the shadow of the hallway. "Hey you!" she said, sudden as a pistol shot. "You! What you doing out of bed?" She stood before me with her arms akimbo before I had pulled my thoughts together.

"I couldn't sleep because of all the noise."

100

"Huh! Well, you get back to bed right this minute! Rose-marie, she says she can't sleep!" Another whoop from the table. Another aide joined in on a chorus of "Light My Fire." The aide confronting me had the singing intonation of the West Indies, and her skin was closer to black than brown. She must have weighed three hundred pounds, and she towered over me. I asked for a sleeping pill.

"You can't have no pills! You should have asked the doctor for sleeping powders. You can't have nothing now!" Framed in the crook of her elbow, the other aides leaned forward to watch. My heart thumped harder than the beat of the song, but I was in it for sure now, no way of retreating.

"Would you mind not making so much noise?" My voice was unexpectedly shrill and scratchy, and for the first time I was afraid.

The aide screamed, "You hush! We got to do something out here, you think it's fun to sit up here all night with you folks, you think we like it? If we don't have some fun, how we going to keep awake? You mind your business, Miss, or you watch out!" She grabbed my shoulder with one huge hand, and spun me around where I stood. Her other hand shot out to catch me before I fell, then pushed at the small of my back. She rushed me down the hall, her sturdy white shoes nipping my bare heels as I fought for my balance. "Don't you let me hear no more out of you!" she said, as she propelled me toward the bed.

Out of the corner of my eye I saw a figure moving fast out of an open archway to the other large bedroom, hiding in a dark corner. I didn't know who it was, but I was glad for the sight of her. Images of drawn knives, wrestler's holds, strait jackets, flicked through my mind in the trip down the corridor, and I clung to the thought that whatever happened, there would be a witness. How easy it would be for the aide to cuff me on the side of the head, blacken an eye, and say I fell. What if she locked me in seclusion for causing trouble, with no mattress, no chair, only the locked door to bang on, and no one to come with a key? But no, I was tossed onto the bed like a five-pound sack of flour, just that light I seemed under the aide's broad hand. My head hit the bedframe when I landed, my elbow cracked against the wall, but the feeling of relief outweighed the pain. I lay crumpled at the head of the bed like a character in an animated cartoon, but the aide spun on her heel, there was her broad back, she was leaving, and I was still alive. Only when I was trembling under the covers did I think that the wraith in the shadows would have been only a poor crazy person, just like me, not a reliable witness at all.

Jeannette Rosetti said, from the darkness, "I don't think the aides should act like that, do you?" in such a mild comforting whisper the tears started down my cheeks. From another bed, Selina Jenks said, "I think I'm going to ask my husband to come take me away from here. They are no good, they don't do nothing for you but give you trouble." There were murmurs from other beds. Almost everyone had been awakened. A few of my tears had fallen onto the sheet by my head, had soaked through, and were dampening the hardened urine beneath. It softened into ammonia fumes rising by my cheek. Like a suicide pulling in lungfuls of gas from an oven, I breathed in that air, counting one-two on the inhale, one-two-three to exhale, until at last sleep came.

Six

In the morning the nighttime shift had vanished like evil spirits. Evelyn was late in waking me, and there was hardly time to wash my face before Miss Pinero called out, "Breakfast, ladies," in the way I was now so used to. It seemed the most natural thing in the world to be called to meals; I wondered how it would seem once again to cook for myself, and eat breakfast all alone. I was by now inured against noticing the encrusted eyes, the fetid breath, the gapes of my fellow patients. Because I still was eating no food at all, save for an occasional overcooked vegetable, my fingernails began to tear like cellophane and my hair was lank. I washed it in the shower after breakfast with a cake of Ivory soap, for lack of shampoo, and then it looked worse.

After medication—I didn't throw it in the toilet when rest-

103

lessness made me irritable, but swallowed it like the most obedient patient—I sat down beside Priscilla in the corridor. I didn't know if she noticed, but I was with her much of the time. Since she had submitted so meekly to Norma June's attentions I thought there was a chance that she missed her, so I would spend time talking to her quietly or not talking at all. Once or twice I held her hand. I usually said things that required no response from her, some piece of news of the ward or a funny remark a patient had made. Sometimes I would talk to her about my feelings on the ward, how sometimes it felt (perhaps it was the Thorazine) as if I was taking a trip inside my head, and meeting people at odd turns. Sometimes fantasy and reality intertwined like ribbons. It was comforting to let these thoughts unwind. I didn't know if Priscilla listened to what I said. Perhaps she didn't hear a word. But if she heard, she didn't seem to find me odd, and I felt free with her.

Priscilla was smiling to herself and nodding her head. "What's so funny?" I asked in a rhetorical way.

Priscilla said, "Don't know." Her words were as clearly spoken as my own. I asked her if she wanted an ashtray, and she said thank you when I handed it to her. Her face was still wistful and empty. The straight straw-colored hair hanging in wisps over her cheeks gave her the look of a young child, and once again I tried to imagine how old she was. She could be eighteen, she could be forty. She was adrift: no name (was it really Priscilla, or Patricia or something completely different? No two aides used the same name for her), no age, no connection to anyone except that strange communion with her mother, and now, so unexpectedly, we were beginning a conversation! I asked her several questions, and to each she gave an answer. I didn't think they were correct answers, they were modest phrases, polite, and just the flicker of concern passed over her eyes, as if she was answering what she thought I wanted to hear. She searched my face to see if I found the answers satisfactory.

"Did you sleep well?"

"Yes, yes."

"Did you have pleasant dreams?"

"Yes. Don't know what kind."

"Priscilla, how old are you?"

"Twenty-nine."

"I've never been in a hospital before Bellevue. Have you?"

"No, just Bellevue, years ago." Then the light behind the blue eyes flickered out, she was quiet, and I didn't ask her anything more.

During the morning I talked to Harvey Barron. He was in his early twenties, still gangly like an adolescent, with a shock of black hair that fell into his eyes, which were large and blue, and innocent long eyelashes that swept up almost to the eyebrows that grew together in a tuft over his nose. I had seen him occasionally on the ward when he stopped by to talk to Phoebe or Evelyn or Jeannette Rosetti. At first I thought he might be a friend or relative come to visit, then again he might be some patient almost ready to go home, and allowed to wear his own clothes—khakis, an Oxford shirt with an open collar. But he talked to the staff with a camaraderie that a patient could not imitate, and several times he was deep in conversation with a social worker. He was the recreation therapist, whose job was to supply us patients with games, activities, and other entertainments. Dropping all pretense of being a patient, I interviewed him like a reporter without a pad—this I could easily do with staff members, they never thought it peculiar. Because most people like to tell about themselves, I garnered full and earnest answers. He had gone to Columbia, he was new to the job, the hospital had invented his position just six months before, and no, he didn't think that he would always be in this sort of work, he didn't know if he was cut out for it, he might try something quite other, perhaps law school. As for his job, yes, he enjoyed it, and yes, he thought he was good at it. I asked him if he thought he reached most of the ladies on the ward, and he said he talked to all of them.

He was a reservoir of good intentions. I asked him about the activities he arranged for the patients, and he told me about ceramics classes, visits to the hospital library, music therapy, dance therapy, woodworking classes, a gym where we might do calisthenics or play basketball; he could supply us with playing cards or Monopoly games or checkers, and he could take us to what he called mass activities in the gym or auditorium on certain nights. I told him that I was delighted to know these entertainments were available. I had now been here five full days, and I had not known they existed until this moment. I asked him why there was not simply a list of activities posted on the wall, so each patient could find out for herself, and he looked surprised. "Why, I don't know, I guess that's a good idea," he said. "You have to understand how new this program is. I've only been here six months. We're still having meetings to set things up. It's bound to be a little confusing in the beginning, but when we get all straightened out, we'll have one of the best recreational-therapy programs in the country. It just takes a little time."

"After all," I said, "since I've been here, I've missed church, I've missed music therapy, whatever that is, and heavens knows what else."

"Oh, well," he said. I saw that I had embarrassed him, and I changed the subject.

"Perhaps you'll tell me when the ceramics class is; I'd like to learn how to work with clay."

He was pleased at that, but told me I would need permission from the doctor. If I obtained off-the-ward privileges, I could participate fully in the recreation program. In fact, he could get me certain materials for use on the ward until I was well enough for those privileges. He had with him a guitar for Jeannette Rosetti to use this morning, for instance. And sure enough, he brought from the office a small battered Harmony steel-string with a crack down the back. I left him besieged by Phoebe and Evelyn, who wanted to try it, to find Jeannette. Her pale face lit up when I pointed to Harvey and the guitar, and soon she was sitting cross-legged on the floor, singing as if she were all alone, with no one listening.

And in truth no one was listening, for the student nurses were busy talking to patients, and aides, social workers, clinicians, nurses were bustling about in the overcrowded corridor wheeling medication carts, conferring with doctors, and attending to the thousand small chores that took up the morning. Two more ladies were going off to state hospitals, and each needed her pocketbook sent up from the property office, they needed to be issued various articles of clothing. Mrs. Weldon, whom I had noticed moaning in sadness my first day here, had spent the week without uttering a word except "Lawd, oh Lawd, oh me," punctuated by sighs. When I had talked to her she had looked at me with pleading eyes and had not answered. Now she stood gloomily like a silent shipwreck in a navy-blue cloth coat that was two sizes too small for her. Her head drooped, her shoulders slumped forward, while she waited to be guided to the elevator. She looked as if she didn't know where she was going, but didn't care.

Leola said brightly, "Hey now, Mama, you put a smile on your face. You say your prayers, now, because the Lord Jesus told me you got a long ways to go before you gets better, and it's mostly your fault, because you ain't trying." Mrs. Weldon looked up for a moment, just a flicker of frightened attention, then her chin sank back on her broad bony chest.

I was sitting with Priscilla while Jeannette played another song, unconscious of how the lyrics sounded here: "'I know where I'm going, I know who's going with me. . . .'" She sang in a clear soprano. The guitar accompaniment was simple but right on the beat. Ineffably sad, she sounded like a waif off the street, and a few minutes later I eavesdropped on her conversation with Miss McMullen. "I kept seeing all these things, like my boy friend in a wine bottle. Isn't that funny, all curled up in a wine bottle. I don't know. All red and yellow, the sun on the glass, I don't know how he fit in there, but it seemed okay to me. You know Peter, Paul, and Mary? They've got a song. I'll sing it, 'He's got a long chain on, he's got a long chain on.' "—I knew that song, about a man escaped from a chain gang in the South—"'Another man done gone, another man done gone.' I thought it was Jesus Christ with the chain on. I saw him crying. I was the Virgin Mary. I thought my boy friend

107

was Gabriel. He didn't look nothing like Gabriel, but I thought he was, because I was all fucked up. Everything was going to be all right, if I could sing right, I had to keep singing, sometimes he would hit me in my head if I didn't sing right. Sometimes when I wanted to see Jesus, he wouldn't come. Lots of times I wanted them to go away, but they stayed with me and I had to play the guitar. If the strings broke it didn't matter. I played a song, like dum de da dum . . ." She hummed a song like a deaf person, hardly making a sound, and what sounds there were turned into a monotone that was ugly on the ear. Her eyes looked far away, and clearly she thought she was singing a beautiful melody. "Do you know that one? I sang that one, and got money, and went with my boy friend, and we walked away. He held on because he was drinking. He kept holding on tighter. Sometimes we had money, though. Sometimes I thought he was Jesus, making the money. I sang this song—do you know this one?—dum de da da . . . " Miss McMullen had that interested observing expression on her face. I wanted to tell Jeannette that she wasn't singing on pitch, that she was making no tune at all, but Miss McMullen said, "That's very pretty." I was disgusted.

Priscilla seemed to be laughing again at some joke of her own, and I thought she might be finding Jeannette's tuneless song amusing. I asked her outright, "Do you like music?"

"Yes," she said.

"If you like to listen to music, I hear there's something called music therapy here. We may have missed it this week, but if you want, I'll ask when the next time is. I think we can sit around and listen to music, and they don't make you do anything you don't want to."

Priscilla said, "Don't like to listen. Like to play. Just like to play music."

I felt goose pimples on the back of my neck. Words, and sentences, and opinion! Why did she leave out the "I"? Did she think that she, the subject, wasn't worth mentioning? Was she here because she had mislaid her self somewhere in the outside world? Except for this omission, we were embarked on a regular, logical conversation!

"What instrument do you like to play?"

"Piano. Like to play piano all the time."

"I used to take lessons, but I never got very good at it, so I just fool around a little with a guitar now and then. What sort of music do you play?"

Priscilla leaned forward and listened to me as if she was trying to understand a foreign language, and was missing some of the words. I asked, "Do you play classical music? Mozart, Chopin?"

Her face relaxed. "Classical. And all kinds. Christmas carols." A pause, and then, as if answering my thought, she said with a slight emphasis on the first word, "I play Christmas carols."

I said, "I'm glad you told me that. I'd like to hear you play sometime. If Harvey could find Jeannette a guitar, maybe he could find you a piano. What do you think about that? There may be one off the ward somewhere that you might be able to use."

Priscilla wrung her hands together. "No, no," she said. "No play piano. No piano." She was on her feet and headed down the hall with her characteristic walk, head ducked, knees knocked together, toes shuffling outward. Her elbows were stuck to her sides, but her hands swung back and forth rapidly, with the fingers stretched out taut.

I said as quickly as I could, "You don't have to, I mean it. You don't have to play the piano." But she was out of earshot.

I spoke to a dark-haired little nursing student about Priscilla. "Maybe she's getting a little better," I said.

"Not really. She's going off to a state hospital soon. That's why her mother has been around here so much. Schizophrenia often seems to affect the whole family. Sometimes the patient does better when she's taken away from the home environment and put in a completely different setting."

I asked Priscilla's age. "Oh, I think she's thirty-three or

thirty-four. That's weird, isn't it? She looks about twenty. Sometimes they look that way, the ones that are very sick." I gave a start as I remembered the policeman who thought I was fourteen. Miss Fitz went on, "It's just my luck that she's leaving."

"You think the state hospital won't help her?"

"No, but she was my patient. I mean I was doing my paper on her. All of us have to choose a patient to do a paper on, we say what we think is wrong with them, and describe treatment and their progress."

"So you're here to study the patients, rather than to treat them."

"Yes, although I think we do them good, you know, paying attention to them, bringing them out." Miss Fitz paused, then jumped with a guilty look on her face. "Oh, you're not supposed to know about all that. I forgot that, well, I mean I forgot—"

"It's all right," I broke in. "You needn't be embarrassed. Sometimes I forget I'm a patient, too. But don't worry, if I ever write a book and quote you, I won't use your name." I said that to be arch, and felt like a fool for doing it. Some book! Some expert! Better to be a nursing student, pinning a patient on paper like a chloroformed moth, labeled. I was so unsure of my premise for being here, I didn't think I could write about it at all. Worse, by playing such tricks with the truth, I was taking revenge on Miss Fitz, who couldn't know how surely the image that she had unwittingly brought to my mind of my scared face in the police station had skewered my confidence in our relationship. Better to play tricks than delve into my mood when I talked to the police.

But Miss Fitz laughed and said, "Thanks. I suppose I shouldn't be telling you about Priscilla, either."

"She sort of opened up a little with me, and I feel fond of her."

"You must be therapeutic for her," Miss Fitz said.

"What?"

"Therapeutic. You must do her some good. You know, she's

a sad case. She's very musical. I've heard that lots of those artistic people break down every once in a while and have to go into a hospital. I don't know if it's true or not, but they say Priscilla used to be a concert pianist."

Mrs. Weldon had gone off alone in a Bellevue car. She had no friend or relative to go with her. She left so quietly I missed saying goodbye to her, and I felt that I had betrayed her.

There seemed to be a larger number of visitors than usual. It was Lincoln's Birthday, and many people were off from work. We patients were more excitable than usual, and there were incidents. Luisa in particular was having a bad day. She had visitors, the man and the woman who had brought her to the hospital, but when she saw them she began to scream in Spanish, "No, no, get away from me, I curse you, you're killing me! *Los maldigo! Alejensen de mi!*" She knelt on the floor and began to beat the linoleum with one slipper. "No! No! *Me estan matando, mi y a mi hijo!*" The woman visitor begged her to get up, but Luisa pulled away from her touch as if she had been burned. "I tell you, you are killing me, you are killing my baby!"

The head nurse worked her way through the crowded corridor and said to Luisa's visitors, "Please, you must leave now. She'll be better later in the week, perhaps, but you aren't doing her any good now. You'll just upset yourselves." The woman began to sob. The man looked grim, took her elbow, and led her away. They did not see Luisa stand up and fling her slipper after them, just before she was put in seclusion once again.

Mrs. Jackson had borrowed Mrs. Foster's lipstick. The red outlined her harelip in two parts, with the scar white down the center. She had a visitor who had come before: a glum balding man in a frayed brown tweed coat that came almost to his ankles. His hair was a faded yellow, and his flat Germanic cheeks were crisscrossed with tiny red veins. The blue eyes were watery and red-rimmed. He might have been a bum, except that his expression was more sensitive and philosophical than that of a bum, and he was stone sober. He held his stained grey felt hat politely in his hand, and did not sit down in the

111

dining room with the other visitors because he wasn't invited to. My friend Helen had come to visit me, and we watched Mrs. Jackson scold him. She shook her finger at him with some violence. He tried to protest, then bowed his head and held his hat against his chest with both hands. There was such a noise of different conversations in the room that it was impossible to make out what Mrs. Jackson was saying, but her vehemence was unmistakable. I hadn't seen her angry before. Little wonder she scoured the bathroom with such fervor—deprived of a spigot to scrub, she turned her energies to this formidable rage.

A stolid patient named Vivian Tursi sat down at the table Helen and I shared. "Some people say he's her landlord, at least she told me that the last time he was here. Maybe he's evicting her, now that she's stuck in here."

Earthalee Emmett leaned over to join us. She was six months pregnant. "Nossir, he's not her landlord. He brought her in here. He's got to be her husband."

"But she told me," Vivian said.

"Up front he may be her landlord. But they've got to be living together. Otherwise, why would he come to visit so often?"

Vivian thought this over for a long time. She was middle-aged, and would have been pretty except for the opaque stupidity of her face. She looked like a cow that had just been poleaxed and was still weaving on its feet. "I dunno," she said. When she smiled, I saw that her front teeth were broken and brown.

"She sure is giving him a hard time," said Earthalee.

Now Mrs. Jackson left off her tirade and sat down abruptly. She looked off into space and started to mutter something. She was not angry so much as querulous now, and she no longer knew the man was standing there. For three or four minutes, she quietly hallucinated. The man stood silent, with his head bent. When the bell rang to signal the end of visiting hours, he moved toward the door. When he passed me, his eyes were filled with tears. They rolled down his cheeks and dripped onto his stained shirt front. He said, "She don't understand. She don't understand nothing."

I put my hand on his arm, and he started. "You did the right thing. Don't punish yourself," I said, taking a guess at their conversation.

He said, "Okay, you tell her. You try to make her see it."

After the last eddy of visitors had squeezed into the elevator, a slender young woman arrived wheeling a record player on a cart in front of her. She plugged it in and waited until some of the ladies had gathered to stare at her. She introduced herself as Mrs. Cobey, the dance therapist. "If you want to hear any music, just pick out what you want. Then, if you feel like moving with the music, if you feel like dancing, you can feel free to do that, too." She had various records: Mantovani, Lena Horne, Harry James. No one moved. She sat on the bench and waited.

I asked her if people usually were so passive. "It varies. Sometimes people start to move, you see some very sick little old lady who hasn't said a word in days stand up and start to move with the music, she can express herself that way. That's beautiful."

I asked her about her background for this work, and she said that before she was married she was with the New York City Ballet Company. "I wasn't a star, just in the chorus," she said. She looked embarrassed that it wasn't more than that, but I thought that was fine, and told her so. I noticed that I was interviewing again, and not acting sick, disturbed, or out of focus; in fact, I was competent. Mrs. Cobey didn't notice, of course, but I wondered if the patients might have picked up something subtle in the mood—were they as sensitive to spies as I?—for no one asked for any music, and no one seemed interested in dancing. The few ladies who shared the bench might have been there because this was where they usually sat of a late afternoon; it was possible they did not notice Mrs. Cobey at all. But they might have waited, quiet as cats, for someone else to make a move. The silence was charged with something like a threat, but maybe it was only that Mrs. Cobey might have no takers, the record player would gather dust, and no old ladies would move beautifully.

Ellis left a card game with Phoebe to say hello. He was in a good mood, his make-up was superb. He was wearing silver eye shadow, mascara, black eyeliner, and on each cheek the most delicate shading of rouge. "Hello, sweet thing," he said to me. "And hello, dear little dancer. Are you going to play some music for us?"

"That depends on you," said Mrs. Cobey. "Choose anything you like."

Ellis thought for a moment, posed with his weight on the ball of his rear foot, his right foot forward, at right angles, like a model. His right fingertips rested lightly on the side of his chin. "Oh, well then, I'll pick something!" he said. He postured again. He was coy. He took *Rhapsody in Blue* from the pile of records. "Oh, how marvelous! Just exactly what I must hear at this *precise* moment!" The music was not the sort to dance to and Evelyn sat looking bored. In a minute she began to giggle behind her hand. Two of the ladies wandered off. Nobody said anything. The music was wrong for this setting, it was almost unintelligible here. It was a white man's jazzy style, romantic and lush. Mrs. Cobey sat with her hands folded, and so did I.

But Ellis saved the situation. He rose to his feet and took a swooping step, arched his fingers over his head like a ballerina. For ten minutes he swung about in the curves of the music, while no one said very much. He was the only one who danced. Mrs. Cobey watched him with pleasure. He began to sweat. The mascara began to run. He dipped and whirled faster and faster. It looked as if he was working hard, and I got the feeling he was doing it as an apology for choosing this incongruous music. For me, it was agony, and I was glad when it ended. No one else volunteered to put a record on, and Mrs. Cobey stayed a little longer with the half smile on her face. I tried to imagine her on stage, with her hair pulled back in just as tight a bun as now, but wearing a tutu, with the stage lights yellow and green and the music of Tchaikovsky. That was another world altogether. Here was beauty of quite another kind.

114

After Mrs. Cobey left, Ellis collapsed in a chair and wiped his steaming face. I asked him why he was in Bellevue. "I was on Forty-second Street, going by a movie theater, in my miniskirt and spike heels, and a woman in a ticket booth called the police. I know she did it, I watched her. I didn't care, I had a couple of pints in me, to keep me warm, you know. I always need something to drink before I go out in my pretty clothes. It's so *cold* out, these nights, if you're wearing such a short skirt. She picked up the telephone. I knew what she was doing, but I just couldn't be bothered to run away. And then the police came. I wasn't doing a thing, I really wasn't."

An aide said, "You was just strolling down the street, not bothering nobody."

"Miss Jessop, I was just my pretty self. I go natural, you know, not like some that wear wigs. I keep my own hair, short, like it is now—I just put a little red in it to go with my skin. May I use your compact for a minute? I'm not going to run off with it."

"I think you could use a little more pencil on your right eyebrow," Miss Jessop said, with a broad wink at me behind Ellis's back.

"Oh, Lord, I do hope they let me out of here soon! My roots are coming in black! This city is no good for freaks any more, do you know that? Just harassment and hard times!"

"It's a shame now. You'll just have to be extra careful the next time you go out for a stroll."

"Miss Jessop, I swear to God I didn't do a thing except walk right by that little glass booth. I wasn't making any trouble."

"Honey, I didn't say you was! I just want to know why a lady would want to call the cops on you. I bet you're so pretty when you're all dressed up, she thought you was her sister."

"You're right! But how could I help it if she didn't like her sister? There's no law against being a freak any more, you know. Mayor Lindsay saw that all the police were out rounding up people like me, and not taking care of crime, and he struck the laws from the books. Now they just psycho you. But I'm not psycho. I like being female, but I'm not psycho. I am what I

115

am, and I know what I am, but the judge gave me thirty days here."

Miss Jessop, Miss Kinney, and some of the other aides who were black had an easier time with Ellis and the more unusual patients than some of the white staff members did. At first I mistrusted this sort of generalization, but I watched carefully the reaction even such a mild and rational patient as I summoned up in staff members, and there were differences. We could joke, we ladies, about some of the funny ways we behaved, we could tease each other, and be teased by some aides; some others must have spent less time appreciating our feelings (and their own) than studying textbooks on our symptoms. They might have cared just as much about us, but they acted constrained. I remembered Miss McMullen, one day, looking at the cover of *The Idiot.* "Now, that's a slick title. I thought I'd tuck it under Miss Hargins' pillow," I had said. There was just the slightest twitch at the corner of Miss McMullen's mouth, but she caught herself in time, she didn't laugh, she didn't really smile. After all, patients aren't supposed to make jokes.

She had said, "I don't know if Miss Hargins is well enough to read very much, but it's a very nice thought."

The black aides weren't so tight or so careful. Perhaps in our unequal society many black women with the natural talents for any profession are shunted instead into work at odd hours and low pay, and so turn a dreary job into an art. In any case, we patients tested the character of those who watched over us, we pulled out the best and the worst in them. Most often, the qualities a staff member needed had less to do with training than with instinct, and with the quality of her own daily life. Black people might live closer to magic than whites; madness partakes of magic, of incantation and ritual. No wonder Miss Kinney, Miss Rivers, Miss Jessop, and most of the other black aides on the daytime shift were more honest with us, as if they too understood that madness might create an order of its own that a person could live with, and never look to Freud for cure.

I was heading for a crisis by Wednesday afternoon. I was used to life on the ward by now. I had done the best I could with it. To preserve my sanity I had spent time as people do in the outside world, doing work, hemming a dress, interviewing patients, making notes. But I lived a parody of life on the outside, for none of it meant anything. Had I swallowed my tranquilizers and sunk into a half-conscious daze, as some of the women did, I still would have been fed three times a day, put to bed at nine, and locked in securely, like a child or an animal. It was that lock that made all this make-work meaningless. I was being locked off from responsibility, and nothing important could transpire here. "But we are alive in here, life still goes on," I said to Priscilla, who nodded idly and plucked at her toes. "Look out the window at those people fighting their way through the snow, packing into the bus to go to jobs—I wonder if they're free out there, and if they know that's important."

Priscilla giggled and grinned. "Free, free, ha ha," she said.

"Okay, I invent the notion that they're free, and I'm not. If they don't know they're free, they aren't, right? If I *know* I'm not free, that I have no control over time, perhaps that's more free."

"Crazy, crazy, no hope," Priscilla said.

I looked at my options. There were the activities designed for patients in occupational therapy: I might make a plastic wallet or draw a picture or play a game of checkers. I had no more than forty cents to put in a plastic wallet, and a picture would only be thrown away, and the checker board was in use. I looked for Sam Buck in the occupational therapy room, but he wasn't there, so I couldn't get him to teach me chess.

Miss Kinney let in through the locked door a man I hadn't seen before. He was heavyset and balding, with bristling eyebrows over the face of a bulldog. His brown suit fit him badly, and the pants broke over his shoes. In one hand he held a clipboard and he chewed on the stump of a cigar.

"Gee, I don't like *him!*" Vivian Tursi said. "I'm going to hide!" She laughed, but backed around behind me, and held up a magazine in front of her face. The man was walking slowly

117

up and down, up and down, making notes on his pad. Patients moved away from him uneasily. From where I sat he looked taller than I knew he actually was, so tall his head was disproportionately small above the slope of his belly.

"That man must be the shock-treatment doctor," I said, although no one had told me any doctor here had that specific position. Here dress, make-up, jewelry, hair style, posture, possessions were either taken from us or obscured by life on the ward and our shapeless, similar nightdresses, but just as a blind man measures distance with his hearing, we learned to pick up information from a squint, a half smile, the pronunciation of a word, the most subtle clues. By contrast, this man in ordinary street clothes, whom I would not have noticed in the outside world, seemed to be wearing signs to his identity. He cleared his throat and angled his cigar in his jaw, and he was unmistakable.

Vivian said, "That's Dr. Soltoff. I don't want him to see me. He wrote my name down before, and I had shock a lot of times." That explained her slow speech and her heavy-footed way of expressing herself.

"How many times?" I asked.

"Eight times. I'm all better, though. I'm going home soon. I used to be like her." She nodded toward Mrs. Foster, who was strapped down in a bed across the corridor. Dr. Soltoff was leaning over her, then making some notes. He spoke to the head nurse and two aides wheeled the bed away.

Before dinner Phoebe yelled, "Miss Kinney! Look on the table! Put out some extra desserts!" The tables were set, and on one of them a large brown mouse was halfway through a serving of cheesecake.

Mrs. Briggs gave a little scream. An aide said, "Oh, now, you just hush. He's just hungry. You have to think of him like he's a pet." She chased him away by snapping a towel at him.

Mrs. Briggs said, "The Mayor should take steps! My lawyer will hear about these living conditions!" But none of the rest of us minded very much. Here a mouse on the table or running along the corridor, or a cockroach in the salad, had no shock value. Even I, as squeamish as any, discovered that I didn't care. A stranger might notice first the vermin and the rodents, but as for us living on the ward, there were other things on our minds. I thought only, "After all, they aren't rats," and quickly forgot about them.

It was the Thorazine, not the mice, that took away my appetite for dinner. I toyed with the canned hash and canned beets, but couldn't eat. My fingernails were beginning to crack and my skin was chapped from the drug, the lack of vitamins and protein, and the dry heat in the ward. I wondered if I would ever enjoy eating again, or if I would ever cook again. I tried to remember the ingredients for a boeuf bourgignon, and the pleasure of putting a casserole in the oven, and it seemed like a great deal of trouble. Like a scientist looking at a test tube I saw my own bored face, and noted the ennui that threatened to steal all profit from this venture. If survival is our only mission, we spend our lives frantically doing more than necessary, overproducing, overemoting, overliving. Perhaps the smart people lie fallow, like fields, just as motionless and still.

After supper I found a pack of playing cards and played solitaire. Out of my childhood came the rules for four different games of solitaire, six, eight varieties. Red on black, odd on even, series of tens, aces high and discard the sevens. I floated on a pleasant Thorazine high.

A new patient was brought to the ward in a wheelchair. She was perhaps twenty years old, with wavy black hair swirling around her face, and clear fair skin. Her cheeks were reddened as if by fever. Her face was intelligent, but the eyes stared transfixed at a point in the middle distance, and her mouth was half open as if her mind was short-circuited just on the edge of a scream. Miss Kearnes and Miss Jessop together lifted her from the wheelchair. They had to put their shoulders under her arms and heave her up on the count of three, for she was tall and heavy. Although her face was stricken with shock, her body was limp, as if it didn't belong to her, and what it did was no concern of hers. She might have been a model for Munch's mad figure trapped in a noiseless cry, the body all sinuous line, made formless by terror. With a thump the girl slipped to the floor.

"Damn," said Miss Kearnes, grunting with the effort to get the girl up again.

"Come on, Faye, try to co-operate," Miss Jessop said gently.

"You get up now, you! Look at that, now," Miss Kearnes said. She poked the girl with the toe of her shoe. "Yell at her until your face is as blue as the sky, and she won't do a damn thing. Deaf and dumb, and stubborn. Get up there, you, cut out your nonsense!"

They wrestled her up like lifeguards dragging a drowning victim. Faye began to moan and shake her head, but her eyes still stared, shocked, at a spot near the door. They got her into a bed in the hallway and strapped her down.

Miss Jessop, gentle Miss Jessop, said in a bemused voice from the other side of the bed, "She didn't fight as hard as I thought she would."

While the two aides were readying a room for seclusion I went up to Faye and put my arm across her waist, and squeezed her as hard as I could. I couldn't put out of my mind how terrifying it would be to lie on the cool linoleum, and far above see hanging in space the grimacing face of Miss Kearnes, with her scowl, her grunts of physical effort, her mustache of sweat. I said, "You'll be okay here, you have time. That's what they give you here. Don't be afraid of the trip." She was wheeled away, the door locked. I didn't think then of how Luisa had welcomed me to the ward. The next day I saw the door to Faye's room open, and the bed stripped. Some time during the morning she had been transferred to another ward or another hospital, and I never saw her again.

Miss Kearnes had brought a puzzle to work with her. A thousand pieces would, when put together, form a mountain scene, a snow-covered stream running through some woods. She set it up on the card table after supper, and started to work it with Eileen, an addict named Fanny, and Sally. The picture was ugly, the colors garish, but this task was right for me. It was soothing and purposeless as solitaire. I was good at the puzzle and worked fast. While the others took the edges, I worked alone on a riverbank covered with blue ice and shadow. Miss Kearnes was impressed at my speed. I was totally absorbed, like a robot programmed to mindless activity. I felt the muscles in the back of my neck unknot. Here was a tranquilizer that affected a nerve center different from the Thorazine.

"Look at her, she's a smart one," Miss Kearnes said. She was having difficulty with the lower left-hand corner. I reached across the table, plucked three pieces, and inserted them without hesitation in that corner. So there, Miss Kearnes! But she did not take offense. "God bless us, look at that. You sure can pick 'em." I was becoming one of her favorites because I was acting like a well person. I was learning fast.

"Thank you for bringing the puzzle, Miss Kearnes," I said. I ducked my head and smiled. I thought of Faye, and Priscilla, and all the patients I cared about, and hated Miss Kearnes, but I knew how to grin and shuffle. "Would you like me to go get the ladies from the dormitory rooms?" I asked, when it was time for evening medication. "Let me go get Miss Hargins, she always gets lost."

The more unctuous I became, the more Miss Kearnes liked me. The more canny I was the less she mistrusted me.

The minimum energy to survive might indeed give a clue to life here, and if here, then life outside, but I was learning that the very minimum took wit and careful attention to detail. At nine o'clock Miss Kearnes ordered us to bed, but tonight I was among the special patients allowed to stay up later. Eileen, Fanny, and I kept at the puzzle for a long time, with Miss Kearnes still working on her corner. I almost fell asleep over the pieces as the hour neared eleven, but I would not give a sign I was tired. At last Miss Kearnes sank into one of the orange chairs outside the dining room and told us to go to bed. I picked up my book and headed down the hall.

The least expected event happened. "What's that book?" Miss Kearnes asked. As I passed she reached out a hand and took it from me before I could think of an excuse why she shouldn't. "*Man's Need and God's Action*," she read out loud. I cursed my cleverness at asking for a book about religion; better to have stayed with Dostoevsky, no one would dream of opening those dense pages. But for a good Irish Catholic, God in a book title was worth a good look.

"You a Catholic?" Miss Kearnes asked.

"No, Episcopalian. It's written by a minister. It's pretty dull." My right hand darted forward like a spastic's to grab the book, but such a move would surely make her clutch it more tightly, and study it page by page. I fought against the muscles of my arm, but they took on moves of their own: grab the book and run, rip it up, flush it down the toilet, hit her, knock it out of her hand. My arm twitched as if someone were tapping a nerve in the elbow, but Miss Kearnes didn't notice. She held the book in her left hand, and with her right thumb she flipped past the front cover, the title page, the first chapter title. I watched in fascination. I heard the rustle of the pages and the thump of my own heart. In my imagination I lived through the first questions: "What's this? Who gave you a pencil? What's this all about?" In some ghastly phantasmagoria I saw phrases from my notes: "Sometimes when I am telling lies I almost believe myself." "Today I figured out how to get rid of my medication." "Sometimes the staff seems crazy." I was relieved that any references to the way I got into Bellevue (or my reasons) were in *The Idiot*, hidden under the blanket on my bed, until it occurred to me that I couldn't explain any of these comments, I couldn't think of a story to cover them, and to a staff member anyone who would write this sort of thing might rate some long-term attention. The doctor would come on the ward, he would ask, "When did you begin having this compulsion to take notes, Miss Barry?" There would be no end to it. I kept my eye on the rough thumb flipping past page 65, page 70.

"I don't know, it's too deep for me," said Miss Kearnes. The pages had stopped turning at the part title for chapter seven. She handed the book back to me. "You get along to bed," she said.

I began to tremble all over. By luck and some intuition two days before, I was spared! I had begun taking notes in *The*

122

Idiot on the inside cover, but with this book, with my pencil poised above the first page, I had stopped short, I had turned the book upside down, and begun writing from the back! Lying in my bed, I tipped the book toward the corridor light and could make out my handwriting. My notes covered the index pages, moved back to front through the text in the ample lower margins, and the last entry was on the back of the part title for chapter seven, directly under Miss Kearnes' thumb! I began to shake so hard the bed squeaked. What a neat escape, how lucky, but could it be that it was more than luck? Could it be that in some magical way I had planned this crisis, as well as its resolution? I was like a playwright who had written his drama in a dream, was caught in the title role and could remember his lines only after he repeated them. There was no telling where the plot would take me next. It must have been one o'clock before I fell asleep. I was afraid to lower my guard, and I was afraid of dreams.

Seven

I woke up out of nightmares, in a sour bad mood. In the shower I shared the stall with Miss Hargins. She washed her hair with Ivory soap, and slicked it down so that it lay in thin rows over her pink scalp. The aide had to remind her to wash away the dried diarrhea that streaked her leg like ribbons. Flo Tamis moved in to take her place, and I was almost crowded out by the huge thighs and vast round belly. "See my beautiful body," she said to me. "Don't you think I have a beautiful body? I had a boy friend once who always liked to show me off to his friends. He was in the army. I would do this." She lifted up each soft white breast with a soapy hand, and bounced them up and down. They were as big as cantaloupes. Miss Kinney chuckled and said, "You put your beautiful body in a gown, Flo, and spare us the sight of it. I don't know that we're up to facing your loveliness this morning."

The shower room was so hot, so steamy, so crowded with damp female bodies, I felt sticky and sweaty before my clean gown was on.

I saw the pack of cards lying on the table, but I was not tempted to try a game of solitaire. I was filled with superstition here, it was the place for it; my close call the night before was a sign that I mustn't give in to boredom. Besides, I now had a meaningful activity to occupy my morning. I had to arrange a way to keep my possessions together, out of sight, and with me at all times. My pockets weren't big enough for two books, my change purse with its pencil inside, my toothbrush and toothpaste, my comb. As soon as the occupational therapy room was open, I asked Miss Pickman if I could sew myself a drawstring bag. She found me some orange plaid material, watched me carefully while I cut out a large rectangle and folded it over. At first permission to use the sewing machine was denied me, but I proved my stability this day by hand basting with great care. When I was done, Miss Pickman stitched up the sides on the machine, then looked at me sharply, and saw that I was uncomfortable. "Well, I guess you can do the rest," she said. "You just be careful." The Singer was old but it worked, and I was pleased with the result, and pleased to be doing it myself. What a responsibility! Once again I began to wonder how I would function when I was released; if such a tiny task was large enough for me to make into a morning's work, how would I manage my own apartment, cleaning, shopping—all the tasks of daily life seemed to require something close to courage to perform. I wondered how it must seem to a patient who had been in the hospital for months, if such a reaction struck me after less than a week. It made sense now that Maxine came back to the hospital each night after her stint as a cocktail waitress, and that Gerta lived here while she went out on job interviews each day.

When the bag was finished I put my belongings in it. I retrieved my comb and toothbrush from under the blanket that served as a pillow, and saw that someone with long black hair had used my toothbrush for a comb.

The doctors were busy on the ward today. Dr. Kegan talked to a steady succession of patients in the makeshift office behind the dining room. Sadie Till pulled at his sleeve as he hurried by, and he looked surprised. "You're still here," he said.

"Doctor, when am I going to have my operation? I'm just in the most terrible pain, and you keep telling me and telling me I'm going to have it, and it never comes time for it. It just hurts so much sometimes I think I'm dying."

"I'm doing the best I can, Mrs. Till," Dr. Kegan said, jerking his eyebrows in an embarrassed way. "I'll see if we can't get it scheduled for the beginning of this next week. Monday or Tuesday for sure."

The corners of Mrs. Till's mouth turned down and she shook her head back and forth. "Oh, Lord, I just don't know, I just don't know," she said. "I can't sit down, I can't lie down, I can't get my rest any way I turn. Give me some pills for the pain, Doctor."

"I'm giving you as much as I can right now, Mrs. Till; any more, and you'll be sicker than you are right now." He ran into his office.

Mrs. Till said to me, "That damn doctor, he don't do nothing. He runs around, and tells you a thing's going to happen, and it never does. He's no damn good."

I murmured something to the effect that he was overburdened with patients, and was doing his best. A moment later, I saw him talking to the head nurse. I strolled over to eavesdrop. He was very angry. "Miss Liggett, why hasn't Sadie Till gone down to surgery?" Miss Liggett shrugged. "I've had that order in for weeks. What do I have to do to get her treated? Would they stall like this if she had appendicitis? Maybe if she needed heart surgery they'd give us some action, and take care of her colon at the same time. I don't care how you do it, but you get her scheduled tomorrow." I'd rarely seen a man more disappointed. "Tell them she's in pain!"

The nurse bobbed her head, "Yessir, yes sir."

Across the room, Mrs. Till was saying to Zélie Briggs, "I been waiting three weeks. Don't you tell me he's done a damn thing! Every time he sees me, he turn his face away. He's ashamed of himself, that's for damn sure." She limped back to the dormitory, still shaking her head.

Mrs. Briggs was trying again to get through to her lawyer. There was another call to her mother, an emotional call, with much fist shaking and sobbing. "I don't know why you don't get me out of here, you can't think I'm crazy, too, you can't." Her dime ran out, and she moved into the social workers' office to place another call. Dr. Kegan walked by quickly, with his head ducked, but stopped short in front of the closed door of the office. He peered through the small glass window and saw Mrs. Briggs huddled around the telephone as if hugging a child. He was oblivious of Mrs. Feeny saying, "Doctor, doctor," at his elbow in a rhythmical reedy monotone. He stared for a few minutes, thinking, then shook his head slowly and sadly, making a clucking noise with his tongue. He might have thought he was alone. Other patients soon assured me that I was not the only one to notice.

"Did you see that!" said Earthalee. "He just don't give a damn what any of us think."

Eileen Thibeau said, "Oh, he's always like that."

"Oh, now, darling," said Miss Kinney tolerantly. "He's not so bad, he's just got too much work to do. Don't you mind his little ways."

To fight the ennui I found creeping over me like a paralytic disease I asked about some of the activities Harvey Barron had mentioned. None of the nurses could tell me when music therapy was, or had been. I saw Harvey talking to Eileen, and asked him again, "Won't you post a list of activities for us?"

He looked abashed. "Well, that's a good idea. I'll have to do that when I get time."

"May I do it right now?" I asked. I could see I was making him very uncomfortable, so I added, "Because of course you're busy, I know you have a big job here. But I have more time than I can use."

"Well, fine, take a crack at it," Harvey said.

And so I made a list, with the aid of various nurses, Miss Pickman, some aides, and Harvey, who sat like a schoolboy who is slow in his lessons as I quizzed him about meeting places and times. "Well, I'll have to find out about that one, I'll get back to you," he would say when I asked him who was in charge of one program or another.

When the list was as complete as possible I found a large piece of white cardboard in the occupational therapy room, some magic markers in purple, brown, and orange, and a broken plastic ruler. By asking two nurses as well as Miss Pickman I got permission to take these materials into the dining room, and spread my work out on one of the tables. I ruled a series of columns, and crossed them with horizontal lines, wrote the days of the week down the side and each hour of the day across the top. As a heading I wrote, "Activities and Other Things to Do," in italic script.

Making the chart was very important to me. It was honest work. Today I knew for the first time that I would be leaving the hospital. I didn't know when, or how it would be arranged, but I knew it was going to happen sometime. I perceived here in two different ways. Sometimes my brain was logical, and avid for details, systems, means. Of course I would be going home! Who would have doubted it? I had planned it from the start! Yet it wasn't until this day, when I started these pieces of work, that I recognized I was practicing for life on the outside.

Patients stood without a word peering over my shoulder. Several told me it was a very good idea. Some wanted to know what I was writing before I could get the words down. Fears of being found out fell away from me, even though as I did my lettering I was noticeably healthy, and the healthier for not minding if anyone noticed. How much time I had wasted here! Days of worrying if my notes would be read, and I had myself put my book in Miss Kearnes' hand! It had been so simple to find the occupational therapy room to make my drawstring bag,

I wondered if it had been those complicated systems and plans that had kept me from going there until today.

There was change in the air here. Harvey had said it, and aides now and again mentioned it among themselves—new programs, new attitudes, new ways of doing things. Attempts to put up screens in the shower room, experiments with group-therapy sessions, and mixing the male and female patients during the day. There was a good chance the information on my chart would be out of date before the day was out, and mislead people. Directly, as I filled in the schedule for dance therapy, I determined to make another chart tomorrow, if the need arose. On a psychiatric ward, patients encourage among themselves the most abrupt twists of motive or logic. I saw no way to chart the future here, but the present was new in an instant, and I could move with it.

Dr. Kegan, on his way out of his office, stopped by the table and asked what I was doing. I showed him the chart, and explained it. "Here, across the top, there's a column for each hour. You can see here, at 12:00, I've made the columns for lunch and the other meal hours very narrow, because we eat so fast." Dr. Kegan smiled and seemed tempted to linger for a moment or two.

Mrs. Briggs said, "Doctor, why don't you put on the chart that all of us get time off for good behavior, and can go home on Saturday." She was trying hard to be in good spirits; I found it almost endearing. Wistfully she said, "You like Miss Barry better than you like me. Maybe you'll let me go home, just to get rid of me." She twisted her lips into a strained, bright smile. Dr. Kegan smiled back enigmatically, and shook his head. With an index finger he drew in the air three zeros. No, no, no. Was he trying to be funny? Impossible to tell. He and Mrs. Jackson, who was gesticulating across the room at a stubborn chair, might have shared some secret crazy sign language, like deaf-mutes, or first-graders with a code.

"Let's see now, you mustn't forget group meetings," he said to me. "Keep up the good work."

Several of the ladies spotted Dr. Kegan, who rarely paused long among the patients, and descended on him from all directions. I put in a request for off-the-ward privileges. "Why, yes, I don't see why not," he said and scurried off.

Zélie Briggs was saying, "You know, he even laughed. Why does he laugh with you?"

"He'll laugh with you if you keep your sense of humor. He's really all right."

During the day I had been smelling something musty and foul nearby. The stench came in waves throughout the day, faint but persistent, and irritating, for I couldn't spot precisely what it was, or where. I looked for Miss Hargins, who usually smelled of feces, but she was nowhere near me. As I worked at the table, the smell grew stronger. When I heard a crisp scratchy sound as I shifted in my chair, I recognized the difficulty at last. The smell did indeed belong to Miss Hargins. It was the reek of diarrhea, but dried into a stale glaze on the gown she had taken off the day before, and which I had chanced to take from the bin this morning. Whenever I sat down the warmth of my bottom activated scents and textures that had passed through the laundry undisturbed. I ran to the shower room as fast as I could, pulling the dress over my head as soon as I rounded the corner of the corridor that cut me off from the view of the visiting male patients, and sure enough, a crisp area some two feet square was smeared with brown. Formidable Miss Hargins! While I sponged off my backside with Ivory soap I muttered about the strength of the weak, how unexpected and pervasive was their influence. It must take special powers for a dotty little old lady to wrap another person in shit, just like that; it took talent.

Swiveled around trying to swab smeared feces off a rump I couldn't see in the scratched metal mirror, I noticed three silent wraiths who stared dumbly at me from the doorless arch to the bathroom—unintelligible and toothless as the Three Grey Sisters, and as cheerless. So much for my charts and drawstring bags, so much for plastic wallets and special privileges. Here work had no value, I had no value. One of the patients stared at my buttocks and slavered, another whined.

"Ladies, turn yourselves around, walk out of this bathroom, and leave me alone," I said. I hid in a toilet stall, a fitting place, to reckon with the trapped hopeless feeling. There was nothing to do with it, it sat there, like a soggy sponge inside my head.

Moments later a nurse summoned me from the bathroom and the other ladies from the dormitory and the corridors, for a large group meeting in the dining room. This must be what Miss Rivers had spoken of my first night here, and what Dr. Kegan wanted noted on my chart. The tables were pushed aside, the chairs arranged in a rough circle, and almost everyone was here—doctors, clinicians, nurses, and aides, as well as patients. One of the clinicians, Miss Eaton, was chairing the meeting.

"We thought it would be a good idea to have general meetings so that you all can talk about life here on the ward, and let us know what you like and don't like about it. Often something might be bothering you that would be easy to take care of, but nothing happens because we don't hear about it, and we can't tell that it's troublesome. Who would like to begin?"

Silence. One of the ladies plucked at her skirt, another began to hum and look at the ceiling. Miss Eaton began again. "Now, I know some of you have some complaints, because some of you have spoken to me about things at other times. Now is a good time to talk about them, to see if other people are having the same problems on the ward."

Flo swung her fat calves back and forth. "We don't get enough to eat. I think we should have snacks in the morning, before lunch. I want bread and jelly before lunch."

Miss Eaton asked, "What do you all think? Do you think there isn't enough food?"

"Oh, Christ," said Phoebe. "That fat slob is always eating. She don't care, she's the last one to want more snacks—if she isn't eating her own food, she's eating somebody else's."

"But I'm a growing girl," Flo said.

131

"Are there any other problems we should discuss?" Miss Eaton asked.

Vivian Tursi said, "There's a problem with stealing. Somebody steals cigarettes all the time."

"And I know who it is," Selina Jenks said. "Everybody know who it is, but nobody make her stop. Two people steal, and everyone know all about it."

"I don't think we should accuse anyone, because so far as I know, no one has caught this person in the act of stealing. But if we talk about it in general, that person will hear how we all feel about it, and will know that she has to stop."

Jeannette Rosetti said, "How is she going to know if she isn't even here?" I looked around the room. Priscilla was here, but wasn't listening. Only Lydie Hargins was missing. "I'll go get her," said Jeannette helpfully, getting to her feet. Everyone laughed.

"That's pretty good," said Phoebe. "You bring her in here, so none of us will know who she is."

"You just sit down, Jeannette. Thank you, anyway, but we can talk about that some other time. Maybe whoever is missing will join us a little later of her own accord."

Phoebe was getting more agitated. She must not be taking her tranquilizers, I thought. She looked like someone high on amphetamines. "Hey, Miss Eaton," she said. "I got an announcement to make. Everybody knows about it, but I got to make it official. Shut up, everybody. Shut up and stop laughing because this is an important announcement."

"Phoebe," Evelyn said, "what are you going to say? What have you got in your mind? You be careful what you say, now."

"I think we'll go on now to the next problem," Miss Eaton said.

"I haven't made my announcement. Shut up, everybody." Phoebe was laughing hard, but her chin was trembling as if she was also on the verge of tears. Her cheeks were bright red. "Everybody, Evelyn and I got married, and now it's official."

"Phoebe!" Evelyn swatted at her, but Phoebe hopped off the table she was sitting on and ran to the doorway. "Catch me, you bitch," she said. She stood panting with her hands resting on her knees. There were tears in her eyes. "You're my wife."

Evelyn yelled, "You hush, now, you damn Phoebe," and tore after her. They ran pell-mell down the hallway, and we could hear them shrieking and tussling in one of the dormitory rooms.

"I want to talk about the lavatory," Mattie Jackson said. "You'll excuse me, but I can't talk so good." She gestured toward her harelip. "I hope you can understand me."

"That's fine, Mrs. Jackson, we can understand you very well," said Miss Eaton.

"The lavatory is filthy and dirty, like pigs use it; nobody keeps it cleaned up. I'm not trying to say it's got to be perfect all the time, but there shouldn't be bowel movement all over the walls and the sinks backed up because toilet paper is stuck in all the drains. That's all I got to say."

"We should all make an effort to keep the bathroom clean," Miss Eaton said. "In fact, we're starting a new program next week that will help us do this. We are going to have different groups in each ward. One group will be in charge of checking the bathroom, another for making sure the beds are made, another for tidying up the corridor, and so on. Then we'll all meet in our groups to talk over our problems with these jobs. Now I want to bring up something that's very important. It has been brought to my attention that some of you are smoking cigarettes in the dormitory. Now, smoking in bed is a very dangerous fire hazard, and it is against the law. Anybody who is doing this should stop doing it, please, or we can't allow smoking at all. Smoking is a privilege, and it mustn't be abused. Are there any questions?"

"I want to ask when I'm getting out of here," Jeannette Rosetti said. "The doctor said I'm supposed to go to Kings Park, but they didn't come yesterday, and they didn't come today, and I want to know when I'm leaving."

"Jeannette, that's a personal problem, and here in the group we're supposed to be discussing problems that have to do with the ward as a whole."

"But they told me I would be leaving, and I got all ready,

133

and I got all my things together, and then they didn't come. I mean, I like it here, I'm not saying this isn't a good hospital, but if I'm going to leave, I don't see why they don't come. You're all very nice, and I don't want you to feel bad that I'm saying this." She was trembling, and blinked away tears.

"I understand that you're upset, Jeannette, and we'll try to answer your question after the meeting. You talk to Dr. Windsor after the meeting, and she will be able to help you."

"Thank you. I'm sorry to louse up your meeting," Jeannette said, sitting down.

The racket stopped in the dormitory, and Miss Sendell left the dining room. A few moments later she returned with the two girls, who sat by the doorway very quietly.

"Nurse, I want to say something." Mrs. Foster was wearing her wig today, and orange-red lipstick, and her false teeth. "I want to say I'm sorry I broke the television set." She grinned and shook her head. "I sure was terrible that day, I sure was. I don't remember nothing about it, but they told me I just threw it down, I was so crazy. I was out of my head, you understand, and I didn't mean nothing by it. Now I'm just so ashamed of myself. I hope you all will forgive me. I had some shock treatment, and I'm better now, thank you, and I'll sure try not to do anything crazy like that again. I'm real ashamed." She winked broadly at Phoebe, who started to cheer and clap. We all joined in a round of applause.

Leola Gibson stood up when the noise had quieted, and began to talk about the noise at night. "Now I know something, and I don't want to talk about it because it's bad, and you all know what I mean," she said mysteriously. "It's what happens at night."

"Ooo, ooo, Gibson!" Phoebe shouted.

"No, I mean it. You know, Phoebe, just what I mean. You ought to know if anybody does."

"Are you crazy? What are you getting at?"

"I'm talking about what goes on in that office late at night, in the night shift. They woke me up last night with their doings, and I know the Lord Jesus made sure I'd wake up, because he was going to make me a messenger to carry the tidings, yes sir, to spread the word about their wickedness. I couldn't sleep last night, no matter how hard I tried, and I sure found out what was going on!" So it was Leola Gibson slipping off into the shadows the night before. She was the witness I relied on.

"What's that the Lord Jesus told you?" Phoebe called out.

"He told me what was going *on* in there, and you know it!"

Someone said, "Let her go on."

"I know the aides do things in that office. I went down to see why there was all that noise, and I got told where to go. They sent me back to bed so fast my head almost got spun off, but I got a look through that door, and I know why they wanted me out of there."

"Go on, there, Gibson, tell what Jesus showed you," Phoebe egged her on, while Eileen and some of the others laughed. Some of the nurses tried not to smile. I was so used to hearing Leola talk about Jesus I hardly heard His name when she mentioned it, but I knew directly what she meant about the aides. In an upside-down way, it made sense: black sisters wouldn't act so mean with no purpose, Leola would reason, so she would try to figure out a purpose that made sense to her.

"Sisters," she said, "I know they pull a bed in there in the middle of the night. Phoebe knows what they do in there, sometimes they let her stay up late and play cards with them. Don't they, Phoebe! They act special with you, so you won't tell on them, and they let you in on it."

Miss Eaton made her face straight and serious. "Just what do they do in that room, Leola?" she asked, with great concern. Dr. Windsor was sitting beside me, a quiet young woman in a cherry red dress.

"Dr. Windsor," I said, getting more upset, "of course Leola's saying crazy things, but that's not important. Don't you hear what she's really saying? Make them stop teasing her. She's trying to account for how tough those aides are at night. You must know what she means."

Leola said, "Jesus told me last night they all was in that room, getting their jollies, that's God's truth, they was in there getting their jollies." Her eyes were very bright and she was wringing her hands with agitation, knowing the whole ward was laughing at her, but she would tell the truth as she saw it, no matter what. "That's what the Lord told me," she said.

"Dr. Windsor, Dr. Windsor," I whispered. "Make them stop. Phoebe is being so vicious, please make her stop."

Dr. Windsor smiled kindly at me. "No, this is all right," she said. "This is fine."

I couldn't believe it. Phoebe was screaming, "Listen to her! She's a nut! Getting their jollies! Woo-ee, did everybody hear that? Who else has seen it? Anybody else hear from Jesus? Don't anybody knock the aides, they're good, you hear me? They're my friends, they work hard, they do a good job! What a life they've got, listening to shit from fucking nuts like Gibson! Getting their jollies! That's rare! Were you in there, too, Gibson? Maybe you went in there with the Virgin Mary? Wow!" She was wound up like a barker at a side show, and Leola looked as if she was being hit.

"I saw it, I saw it," she kept saying, but nobody was listening. They were laughing, and cheering Phoebe on.

"Dr. Windsor," I said, with the tears rolling down my face, "what's going on? Am I crazy, Dr. Windsor? I feel as if I'm listening to someone speaking a foreign language, and nobody can understand except me. I tell you, I know what she's saying. Not about the bed in the office, but about how bad the aides are, how they chased her away, that was true, Dr. Windsor. Tell me, please, am I crazy? *Am I crazy?*" I couldn't stop crying. As if the clock flipped back to the night before I saw the huge face above me and felt again the terror as I was whipped around by hands as big as a prize fighter's, and I wondered if I would ever be able to describe that fear that I felt then, that Leola had picked up, too, just us two.

"Don't worry, it's all right," Dr. Windsor said. "This is just fine." Paranoia took me over entirely.

"What are you trying to pull?" I asked. "If you don't care about complaints, why are you having this meeting? Are you taking notes on us? Are you taking notes on Phoebe? Are we in a zoo, for you to watch?" But I kept my voice sweet and soft, with the tears falling into my lap with little plopping sounds, and Dr. Windsor, who was watching Phoebe intently, said, "It's important for people to get their feelings out."

Miss Eaton cut through all the catcalls and hooting by saying, "All right, now, if there are no other comments, we'll close this meeting." No more was said about the aides making noise at night.

The ward meeting was a fraud, I should have known that. Selina Jenks had sat through it half asleep; she knew what was going on, but I had fallen for it. Now I couldn't stop crying. Leola wouldn't hurt anybody, I knew that, and she shouldn't be laughed at. What was wrong with me, that I could talk to Leola, and not begin to get through to Dr. Windsor? She wasn't much older than I, she worked long hours. She cared about her patients; and yet she was more alien to me than the spookiest psychotic on the ward.

I was tempted to call Michael Allen on the telephone, or Helen, but I held back. Partly, I thought with New England rigor, because I had gotten myself into this fix, and it would mean nothing if I could not get myself out; partly because my difficulties were here, on this ward, as close as my own thoughts, and although there might be comfort from outside, all the work had to be done on the spot. In total misery I thought in turn of murder, suicide, and forcible escape. In the hour before supper I tried to reason with myself, and unexpectedly I fell into a sound sleep.

Zélie Briggs woke me up, saying, "I called the lawyer, and I'm getting out of here. Just you wait and see. The lawyer is getting a writ of habeas corpus, and I'm getting out of here. That will show that doctor that I meant business!"

At supper I sat with Leola. I was confused by the strength of my feelings when she had begun to speak at the ward meeting.

Maybe I was better off talking to her than to a doctor, after all. Surely I felt on the defensive, for I started out taking a reporter's detached tone. I asked about her family.

"There's my husband, Beauregard, and there's Clarence, he's six, and Beauregard Junior, he's four. Roxanne is three."

"I saw your husband coming to visit you the other day. He's a handsome man."

"I used to think he was, but he's a sinner, and I'm not going to live with him any more. He drinks liquor, and smokes cigarettes, and he won't listen to the Lord. I told him Jesus said he has to stay out of my bed, but he won't listen to that, either."

I asked her why she was in Bellevue. "I was a crazy woman! I thought it was Armageddon, right here and now! I was running around to all the neighbors, and telling them about the Day of Judgment. Wasn't that something! In the middle of the night I was running around in my nightgown, banging on people's doors! Say," she said, narrowing her round bright eyes at me, "you know, you sound just like a social worker." I froze. "That's something I just noticed about you."

"I don't know, I'm in here just like you," I said.

"It's just a feeling I got. Sometimes the Lord talks to me. Maybe it means you're getting out of here soon."

After supper I wanted to exercise my new privileges. "You can come to ceramics class if you want," Harvey said. I followed him through the locked doors, past the elevator and down another long corridor.

The room where the ceramics class was held was, like the occupational therapy room on the ward, crowded with materials of all sorts, pleasantly disordered, like an attic. Along two walls were shelves holding patients' handiwork in various stages of completion. There were ashtrays, mugs, clay baskets, some formed on the wheel, but most made by simpler, cruder methods. Harvey showed me how to wedge the clay, and how to flatten a smooth slab to form a cup with it. He showed me how to make a long snake of clay and coil it around on itself to make a dish. I worked with complete absorption. The clay was cool, and it had texture. For days there had been too little in my life to touch, pick up, feel. I knew the shapes of my paperback books, my comb, my toothbrush, my drawstring bag, for I had spent time holding them; only now did I appreciate how many other objects one touches in ordinary daily life that I missed here.

On the ward, all my senses had become attenuated in a state of slow starvation. There were only so many colors to see, most of them neutral greys and browns; I now appreciated the harsh bright paint on the dormitory doors, and would have wished for chartreuse and crimson as well. The eye hungered for variety, and missing it, saw even less than it was given. As the routine of the ward became more familiar, even what sounds there were —the drone of female voices, broken by occasional cries of laughter; the swish of slippers on linoleum; the gabble of a distant television set or record player; the clatter of plastic dishes and spoons three times a day; the flushing of a toilet—these sounds melded upon constant repetition into a sort of white noise that was irritating rather than refreshing. I was unaware of this attrition of my physical sensitivity until this night, and so also unaware just how much of my sense of my own being was determined by my responses to my immediate physical environment. Whether one prefers blue to yellow or the scent of roses to the scent of baking bread seems a minor matter until one has gone without the choice for a time; just as one's old roles in the world grow dim in outline so whatever part of the self affirmed by the senses tends to shrink away, and one explores inner, new ways to assert one's individuality. To spend even this short time back again in sensuous activity was to come upon myself unexpectedly, as if after a long journey.

The satisfying "thok" of the clay on the board, the solidity and the dampness, gave me a special pleasure. I rolled out a slab of clay and cut it with a knife into a long square cord, and coiled it around like an Indian basket. The neck was narrow, there was a lip around the edge.

It felt normal being off the ward. I forgot that I looked as scruffy as any patient, and was still wearing a hospital dress. To my relief I felt competent. It was natural after all to begin a task, to follow it through, to finish it. The time passed quickly, and I was disappointed when it was time to go back to the ward. That evening Miss Kearnes again brought out her puzzle, and I set to work on it with several other patients. By now I was one of Miss Kearnes' special pets, and I knew I would probably be allowed to stay up later than usual. At eight-thirty the cry went out, as usual, "Medication, ladies!" but I ignored it. I wondered what would happen if I kept mum; I could see that the medicine on the cart was in liquid form, and there was no way to get away without swallowing it. But perhaps tonight I would be lucky, and they would overlook me.

One by one the ladies shuffled up to the cart. Now that I knew them, they did not look drab and unattractive. Belle Grumbacher, adjusting her hearing aid, Luisa, with her long braid absolutely neat, Mrs. Foster, Eileen, Jeannette Rosetti, Phoebe, Leola Gibson, pregnant Earthalee, Sadie Till—they were all my friends. Only Mrs. Feeny, the desiccated little figure Luisa had so persistently attacked, stood off suspiciously from the rest and glared.

"Come get your medicine," Zélie Briggs said in a friendly fashion, as if she had never considered it anything but a privilege to stand in this line four times a day.

"Umm-um," I said, adding another section to the mountain stream. Ten minutes later Miss Kearnes was yelling at stragglers in the dormitory to come to the cart, Flo Tamis was complaining at the taste of the medicine, Irene Tompkins was swinging high on her paraldehyde—and the cart was rolled away. I had escaped. For another half hour I was ignored. "She still working on that puzzle?" Miss Kearnes said to another nurse, over my head. "You, all right now, you get to bed."

I had outfoxed myself. I lay with my eyes wide open, staring at the ceiling. Better to be drugged into sleep than not to sleep at all. An hour went by, then another. Every muscle ached, my elbows and knees were chafed by the muslin sheet as I turned first one way, then another, and listened to the nighttime moans

140

of troubled sleepers, heard the aides' muffled voices down the hall. At midnight I padded down the hall to find the head nurse. I knew better by now than to be caught by an aide.

"Dr. Kegan said I might have some medicine to help me sleep if I needed it," I said.

"No, you can't. I don't have the authorization."

"Would you look and see if you do? He really said he would leave permission for me to have some sleeping medicine."

Miss Foley made a desultory pass at a stack of papers on the desk in the nurses' office. "No, nothing here. You go back to bed."

I gave up. "May I have my nighttime medication then? I missed it somehow before bed."

Miss Foley glared. "What do you mean, you missed it? You get right into bed this minute." She followed me down the hall to my bed, scolding me all the way. The more she talked, the more witchlike she looked to me. Her nose seemed to curl down over her lip, her chin grew sharper. I began to wonder if I was hallucinating. I kept a penitent expression on my face, and figured that the energy of my anger was reshaping her face like clay.

"Coming for your medicine when you're called is part of your treatment," she said.

"Isn't it lucky it was just a tranquilizer, and not insulin or digitalis or something that might have mattered."

She looked sideways at me. "You're a bad girl," she said. "It's your fault." So, at last, I was a responsible party! "You could get in a lot of trouble for this," she said.

I could get in trouble! The rage welled up again, and my helplessness only aggravated my feelings. I made myself say, "I'm sorry, Miss Foley."

"You just be grateful I'm not going to tell the doctor."

I said, "My medication is Thorazine." She whirled on me in triumph just before she headed for the nurses' office. "I'll look it up, thank you! I never trust the word of a patient!" When she returned with the Thorazine I had made myself very calm.

"Thank you very much," I said. I was so eager to cover my wrath I was almost talking baby talk.

"That's all right, dear," Miss Foley said. "I'll forgive you this time." She squeezed my hand. "Just don't do it again." When she was safely out of earshot I said into the air, "Why don't you let me do your job, and you be the patient. You can have my smelly bed." I knew she couldn't hear, but I felt better.

Selina said, "They're all bitches." I saw the glow of her cigarette in the darkness.

Jeannette woke up. "Look," she said, "I don't want to make trouble. I don't like trouble, but you know."

"What you talking about?" Selina asked.

"The cigarette."

"What? You want a cigarette?"

"No, you know, about the rule. At the meeting they said, no smoking in bed. I just want to do the right thing." Because the foot of Jeannette's bed was backed up against the foot of mine, I could feel her movements, just as Evelyn could no doubt feel mine in the next bed up. From the gentlest quiver of the metal headboard I could tell that Jeannette was trembling with agitation. "I don't like to make trouble," she said. The conversation was difficult.

"Christ," said Selina. "What the fuck you talking about? Don't you get on my back."

"I was just trying to help," Jeannette said.

"You mind your own business."

"I don't know when to do what they say. Sometimes I do what they say and I'm wrong, sometimes I do different and I'm wrong."

"I know," I said in full sympathy. "You just have to take your chances." I thought about Leola and how she had misjudged the ward meeting, and how I had, too. Leola had recovered from Phoebe's attack in a matter of minutes. "Some people can get blown apart and get themselves back into one piece again. I guess you don't have to be responsible for what other people want you to be. You can fight back, or at least you don't have to give in."

Most of us have the kindness to hide our best nature at least part of the time, but Jeannette was totally kind always, and totally vulnerable. She was incapable of malice, and so Selina and Phoebe could spare her no respect.

"I think I'm going to Kings Park tomorrow," she said.

"Do you like it there as well as here?"

"It's not bad, I guess. Some of the people are nice, but the place you stay isn't as good as this. I just want to be settled down, you know what I mean? I'd like to know what's going on."

I didn't know how to answer that, so I wished her luck and we went to sleep.

Eight

On Friday patients were leaving. Ladies I had no idea were ready to go home were sitting around with their coats on from soon after breakfast. Vivian Tursi was dressed up in a knit suit that dipped under her buttocks tightly and outlined rolls above her girdle; she was impressive at breakfast. There seemed many fewer of us at that meal, but it was not true; there were no actual departures until after ten, when the staff was on the ward and forms were ready to sign.

During showers Evelyn asked me when I was going home, and when I told her I didn't know, she seemed surprised. "I bet you go home soon. Dr. Kegan's got a crush on you." Mrs. Briggs, stepping into the shower I was stepping out of, looked gloomy. "I wouldn't put my trust in that fool. Get yourself a good lawyer. I fully expect to be released by noon."

Outside the shower room Miss Jessop was sitting beside a

wagon that held some black plastic combs (without points) and some odds and ends of make-up. There was loose powder in a dark orange shade; some stubs of lipstick, purple, tangerine, and cerise; a tawny yellow eyebrow pencil. The ladies lined up to use the roll-on deodorant in turn. It had no effect on that acrid odor I had noticed in the shower room.

I asked Miss Jessop if I might use the eyebrow pencil, and for lack of a proper mirror (that was not available to us even under the eye of an aide) I applied it in front of the steel mirror over a basin in the bathroom. I asked why there was no dark brown or black pencil, as there were few enough blondes on the ward. Miss Jessop said, "They get stolen, honey. I just can't keep them on the cart."

I tried out my new off-the-ward privileges as soon as the beds were made. I was giddy with self-importance. I yelled out, "Snack bar!" as loudly as I could. I was immediately surrounded by the ladies. Eddie and Bill were visiting, and stood off from the rest, uncertain if I would count them in. All my exhilaration faded as I listened to the various demands. They may have asked for candy or cigarettes, but their voices penetrated like the squawks of angry birds, and their faces looked to me as threatening as a circle of outthrust, gaping beaks. My voice was a chirp. "One coffee? Light or black? What did you say your name was? You want to change that to tea? What?" I was forgetting the orders as soon as they were thrown at me.

Mercifully, Vivian Tursi appeared at my elbow with a stub of pencil borrowed from a nurse, and a scrap of paper. "Write it down. You have to write it down like this." She made a three-column list. "Put the name, and then what they want, and then the money." I collected the change, and with her help filled in the columns like an accountant.

Bill said, "The fellows on the other side would sure like it if you got some stuff for them. There's only one guy with snack-bar privilege, and he never feels like going." The men who visited regularly told us tales about O 7. The aides spent little time with the patients, and didn't enforce even those rules the patients tried to impose on themselves. "None of the beds get made, and nobody cares. Nobody goes down to the snack bar, and we don't even have a television set." Coming from N 7, of course I couldn't inspect the men's dormitories or their bathroom to see if they were as foul as Bill reported; nor could I check whether stealing was that much more widespread than among the ladies, but judging from the number of men who visited whenever the doors between our wards were unlocked, they considered the part of the corridor that formed our day room a country club, even after our television set was broken.

The crowd that gathered on the men's side was more vociferous than the ladies. My list grew longer. Each order had to be queried: filters or kings? large Coke or small? Vivian, though slow, was steady. Our list was completed, an aide unlocked the purple door. Vivian asked her twice to tell Mr. Tursi to wait if he came by to pick her up, that she would be right back. The aide accepted that without seeming to notice that there was really no way she might avoid coming right back, short of a full-scale escape.

Going down in the elevator was enough to make me feel shaky. Having no aide with us was almost like being free. Being on the inside of my hospital gown and slippers, I didn't have to look directly at them, and I could pretend that, like Vivian, I was going home today.

The lobby was tall and vaulted, with 1920's Byzantine trim: tessera inserts on the ribbed ceiling, arches over the windows, and massive columns for support. Visitors' footsteps rang on the stone floor. The snack bar was brightly lit and tawdry, tucked in a corner like an afterthought. It offered sandwiches as well as cigarettes and coffee. We joined a ragged line of aides getting coffee, visitors waiting to see doctors or for visiting hours to begin, and other patients, like us, who invariably held handfuls of change tightly. The man told us the jelly doughnuts had run out, but there were three crullers left; he was out of Pall Mall regulars, but he had kings. He had no Danish, and no candy bars at all. Vivian and I began to fill in alternatives on the list. Because some twenty individuals had asked for twice that number of items, we had to write down every substitution. Behind

146

us people in line grumbled. "Never mind them," Vivian told me. "We've got a right to bring our business here."

The elevators were being replaced with more modern ones, and the process was taking months. The one car that worked had no button with which to summon the operator: one tapped on the window for his attention. Almost ten minutes passed before the car arrived, and there was barely room for the crowd that had collected. Four policemen in uniform caught the doors just before they closed. One held a paper cup of coffee. He said to us, who were near the door, "This is a police emergency. We have to use this elevator. Get out." As the doors closed, they chuckled. While we waited fifteen minutes for the next car, Vivian thought this through. She said, "What do you think? I don't think there was a real emergency."

On the ward we distributed the food. I started to panic. Nothing was coming out right. I owed patients nickels and quarters in change, but I held only dimes. Some of the men were disgruntled at the substitutions in their orders. I couldn't concentrate on my list. Trying to sort out faces, names, money, and goods, I could cope with none of it. Vivian completed each transaction one step at a time. I revised my opinion of her.

When medication was handed out, I took my Thorazine. After the morning's adventure I didn't mind a tranquilizer. Leola was sobbing by the cart, but her expression was ecstatic. "Jesus talked to me last night. He told me He wanted me to take my medicaton, Miss Sendell. I spit it out every time, because I was misguided. But now I want to do what the Lord tells me; I don't want to be wicked. Miss Sendell, give me mine right now. Let the last be first and the first be last, that's what He said. Praise be, sisters, you all got to take your medication now." A half hour later, Leola was drifting around the ward in slow motion. The ecstasy was transmuted into the most gentle and beneficent smile, and for fifteen minutes at a time she stopped talking.

Sadie Till had at last been taken off in a wheelchair for her operation. The car came from Central Islip and took away Miss Hargins, who complained as they bundled her into a coat.

Vivian's husband came, and Vivian said, "Lots of luck, now," several times to everyone on the way out.

I took a nap before lunch. The dormitory was empty except for Selina Jenks. She was lying in bed, smoking. She said, "I called up my husband to come to get me. God, I missed him so. I don't have to stay here no more." A few minutes later she stubbed out the cigarette on the bedframe and hunched the covers up to her chin. As I was falling asleep the creaking I had heard each night began once again and Selina's blanket lifted and fell to its rhythm; what would have nonplused me a week ago seemed natural enough today. "So that's what I heard," some character said inside my head, before the dream spun me off into some terrain far from the ward.

When I was talking to some of the male patients after lunch it was evident that my panic of the morning had been forgotten if it had been noticed at all. When everyone has problems, no one must pay. Apologies, social lies, and other disguises for our own failings are as irrelevant on the ward as, it began to dawn on me, they might well be outside. The men were friendly enough, and Eddie was eager to teach me the chess moves that Sam Buck, who had gone off to another hospital, had taught him. Bill asked me if I was going to the Sweetheart Dance that night in the auditorium, and reminded me that it was Valentine's Day. I promised I'd see him there, for I'd gotten off-the-ward privileges.

"Dr. Hunter says I'm too sick to go, myself. I feel real bad about it. I heard some of the guys talking about it, and I wish I could get well fast."

"What does the doctor say?"

"I'm depressed."

Mrs. Feeny poked her weasel face at him. "What's your name?" she asked in a reedy voice. She had been very quiet since she arrived, like many newcomers, and I was interested to hear what she had to say.

"Eddie," he said. "Eddie Polanski."

Mrs. Feeny sucked her lips over her gums. "And an American. You're a nice boy. Better than some here. There aren't

148

enough Americans in this place. The Jews and the P.R.s, that's who run things. And the niggers, too. Just look around this hospital. Look who gets the special treatment." By now she was whispering just inches from my ear. "It's the P.R.s. Look at who's working here." She nodded at Miss Kinney, who was not Puerto Rican, but black, and Miss Pinero.

"You're certainly American," I said. "You remind me of some people I've run into."

"Look at the doctors. Look at *him*." She tilted her head at Dr. Kegan across the corridor. "You have to be careful who you talk to these days."

Mrs. Briggs caught only this last speech and was eager to add her comments. "That fool! I'll tell you what sort of individual he is! He lives in Great Neck, Long Island, with a stupid wife and three children. Every night he must sit on the train and congratulate himself on his success! He must take vacations in Florida, on the family plan. He has no taste."

This seemed less than fair. It more likely described the past that Mrs. Briggs didn't care to talk about. I said innocently, "You come from a more aristocratic background."

Mrs. Briggs might stretch a point, but she wasn't a liar. "Not precisely, my dear. However, I did marry well. I married very well. And I have known people of influence; I am a writer. I've written articles for *Esquire*, I had a column in the *World-Telegram*—that was some time ago, you're too young to remember—but I have many friends. I count Tennessee Williams among them. Yes, you might say that I have pretensions to something better than that ill-bred fool. You know, there is a certain sort of Jewish person . . . "

Mrs. Feeny asked suspiciously, "What country are you? Where are your people from?"

Mrs. Briggs was caught off guard. "Are you inquiring about my ethnic background? I would say that I am, ah, an American." Mrs. Feeny beamed. The two of them, unwittingly both enemies and allies, walked off down the corridor deep in conversation, leaving me to wonder if it had been chance that Luisa had singled out Mrs. Feeny when she pulled her frizzy hair.

Dr. Kegan hurried past on his way to lunch. He said over his shoulder, "Miss Barry. You're going home tomorrow."

"I can really leave! You mean I'm all well?"

Dr. Kegan gave a cryptic look. "I'm going to talk to your minister again. I'm going to suggest to him an outpatient clinic for you, one that should cost you very little money. There may be a waiting list to get in. If there is some work in the parish office for you to do, I think you should do it." This was a long speech, and by the time he was done he was almost to the locked door. He didn't give me time to answer, but put his key to the lock, and slipped out to the corridor beyond.

"That man is always in a hurry," Miss Kinney said. "You watch, he's going to get a hot dog down on the corner from the man with the hot-dog wagon. He don't even take the time to sit down in the cafeteria."

"Miss Kinney! Did you hear what he said? I'm going home!"

"Well, how about that! That's *good* news!" I was congratulated all around as if I had done something fine. I said, "I'm pretty healthy." The rush of homesickness and relief was so strong I forgot that I wasn't really a patient here. And I had done something fine. I had gotten through a week here, I was getting out (I was not quite sure how), and I was the better for having been here.

Mrs. Briggs had come back down the hall to try a telephone call to her lawyer. When I saw her face I wished that the aides would stop talking about my release. Mrs. Briggs, Phoebe, Evelyn, Mrs. Foster—there was no telling when they would get out. Belle Grumbacher was going home on a weekend pass, and I switched the conversation over to a listing of her children and their ages. It took effort because Belle had dropped her hearing aid on the floor and it no longer worked. She wore it in her ear anyway, as if a dead hearing aid was better than none at all. We shouted back and forth. In moments the news of who was leaving and who had weekend passes had been forgotten or put aside. News died quickly on the ward. There were newer, more personal matters in the life of each patient than the events in someone else's life.

At two o'clock Miss Kinney took Earthalee, Leola (whose new enthusiasm for her medication had been noticed by Dr. Windsor), and me to the beauty parlor. It was past the locked door down the corridor, near the ceramics classroom. It in no way partook of hospital atmosphere. It was a beauty parlor, sure enough, with vinyl-upholstered armchairs with hair dryers attached, counters cluttered with combs and curlers, and over them large mirrors that reflected customers and operators in multiple dumb show. Around the walls were photographs of hairdos cut from magazines of the trade. One sheet showed six black girls with straightened hair in waves and ringlets. Some hand-lettered placards said, "Black Is Beautiful!" and pictures drawn by patients decorated the walls. The room smelled, like any small-town beauty parlor, of plastic, shampoo, wet hair, and cheap perfume. The two operators were elaborately coiffed in styles like those in the pictures on the wall.

When I took my place in a chair to wait for my turn, and saw my first real mirror in seven days, I thought of all the mirrors I used on the outside—one from my pocketbook for putting on lipstick, a couple in my apartment that I glanced at as mindlessly and doubtless as frequently as one checks a wristwatch. I thought of catching glimpses of my reflection in store windows as I walked along the street. In a typical day I figured some fifteen glances at a mirror were not unusual. Fifteen times a day I used to remind myself what I looked like, I checked the effects of late hours or a nap, of a happy mood or a low one. Here in Bellevue I had seen only the haziest blur of myself in the scratched mirror above the sinks some two or three times since I'd been here. The outlines were so dim I'd given up looking for my image in them early in the week, in fact hadn't made a conscious effort until this morning. By my arithmetic I'd missed in this week some hundred images of my face and figure. Now I saw myself sharp in these clear glass mirrors, and I was shocked. I had lost at least five pounds, and my cheeks were hollow. My hair was longer than I remembered it, and a somewhat darker color. My eyes seemed smaller, and deeper set, and my skin was without tone. A dead bland little face atop a body with no shape in the hospital gown. My eyebrows were lightened, not darkened, by the yellow pencil I had borrowed this morning from the aide. I had drawn the line a good half inch off the natural arch by mistake, giving the upper half of my face a piquant and foxy look. My lips I had remembered as pink, but they were white. The overall expression was sad and shy. During the week, in my mind my distinctive features had blended into a generalized female face.

The operator put a telephone book on my chair so that my head would reach back far enough for the shampoo. In the mirror I saw that everyone in the room was a head or more taller than I. I was the size of a child. It was a rediscovery so abrupt it seemed news to me. This week, I had lost my size and I cared about myself nonetheless. Now, here I was again!

The beauty operator promised to make me particularly pretty. "We'll make you look special for the Sweetheart Dance tonight." While she put in the rollers I asked how she happened to be working at Bellevue. "I came looking for a job as an aide, but they had this job open and I took it. I used to run a beauty parlor, but I gave it up. I wouldn't work anywhere else. There's satisfaction in it. It's nice to see how pleased the ladies are to see themselves all fixed up. It gives a person a lift, after all, when you're not feeling good."

Leola said, "I been here before. This lady knows just how to do things right. She's doing the Lord's work. This Earthalee, she's something else again." The medication was wearing off.

Earthalee gave a sigh. "Shut up now, Gibson."

"I told you this morning I was sorry for bothering you yesterday, and you turned your face away from me. I asked you to forgive me, Earthalee, and you didn't do it. I asked you not to hold a grudge against me, and you're doing it, I can see it plain. You're in the Devil's hand, and you're saying nasty things about me behind my back. And after I apologized to you. You sure aren't a Christian. Do you think that's right, Barry, that she should act like that? I prayed for her, because I was feeling the glory of the Lord flowing through me, and she won't forgive me."

Earthalee folded her hands over her stomach, which swelled up almost perfectly round under her robe. She looked half asleep. Her eyes were heavily lidded, and revealed that mood of blank introspection common to pregnant women. Leola's voice grew shriller and shriller as she got no response. Earthalee shifted her weight and, slow as a turtle noticing the sun, she blinked and said, "Leola, I done nothing to you. There ain't nothing I can forgive you for, because you ain't done nothing to me. You're doing something now, though, you're making me sick of the sight of you."

Leola's eyes turned into slits. "Sister Earthalee, you're an evil woman. God's going to put a curse on you, for sure. I never did like you much."

The second operator heated up a little stove on the counter. When it began to smoke she pulled from it a heavy iron comb, now glowing red hot. The thick tines of the comb came within an eighth of an inch of Earthalee's scalp, there was a hiss, the hot smell of singed hair, and a lock stood up straight as if pasted onto thin air. The woman worked quickly. The stove with the comb in it began to glow an alarming red. "Bella, you unplug that thing!" the first operator cried out. "We get the most no-good broken-down junk in here, it's a risk to your life to do your job. I burned my hand on that stove so often I don't hardly feel it any more when I do it again. I know I shouldn't complain. The hospital's short of money, and all this is donated, secondhand."

Michael Allen had promised to visit today, and I was nervous. It was well past visiting hours, and just like Vivian Tursi this morning, I wondered if I would be found. On the ward there were no choices to be made; one was not accountable. My new privileges put me on the spot. Would Michael miss me? Would he be cross that I would pass up a visit from him just to have my hair set? I knew he was busy; he wouldn't be pleased to make a wasted trip. But maybe Dr. Kegan had taken him into an office to talk about my future. I fidgeted in my chair and asked the operator not to bother to comb me out; I would do it myself back on the ward.

"Oh, darling, you sit right here. Don't worry, your visitor's going to find you. They'll bring him right down here. You want to look pretty for tonight. Don't you look, now. I'm going to turn your chair around so you can't see the mirror. I want you to have a nice surprise."

Leola was under the dryer, and Earthalee was all done, her hair slicked back from her forehead and puffed up in little curls behind her ears, so the second operator was free to assist. The two women made me their special project. They brushed and combed and sprayed, they pinned and crimped, they made some spit curls, they waved the back.

A nurse came by and said, "I've got a visitor here for Barry. Earthalee, you want me to take you back?" Earthalee preferred to see how I came out. She and Father Allen joined three aides who stopped by to say hello to the hairdressers, and who stayed to offer advice and opinion on my progress. I was rigorously warned not to move an inch, or I'd ruin their work. I could see Michael out of the corner of my eye. He looked uncomfortable, as if he was unsure of what he had done; had he known the staff members were so kind, he might not have abetted my efforts to fool them. What right had a healthy girl like me to take up their time and their affection?

"Just hold still now. We're making you look like a princess. Earthalee, now what do you think of that? Don't peek, Miss Barry. You hold your head still. I'm going to find you something pretty to put in your hair." The operator searched under the counter for a special box from which she took a piece of yellow ribbon, somewhat wrinkled, but carefully folded. I could feel her threading it through my hair and tying the bow. "Now look at that!" she said. There was a chorus of exclamations. It was a success! Michael looked more uncomfortable.

I wanted to tell him that I did belong here, after all; partly because as a patient I made a contribution here. I saw the ward as a closed system in which each patient and each staff member had his own particular effect, responding from moment to moment to shifting demands. I took part in ward life, and I had my place. Earthalee shucked off lethargy to suggest that the ribbon be moved over the left ear; Leola forgot to curse her and agreed. Each of us, in our separate ways, was important; even the least responsive had a place. If Belle Grumbacher, deaf and depressed, stood stolid as a cow under Evelyn Howard's harangue, Evelyn Howard was then able to spare one of her candy bars for Flo Tamis. In the closed economy of the ward, no gesture was lost.

I thought about the chart I had made, and about its use, and some other patient, at another time, making it over and listing the new activities just as I had done. I thought about what a variety of experiences lay ahead, just outside the ward, and how differently I might feel about them. If I could manage here, I might survive on the outside.

It was impossible to say this to Michael at this moment. I almost wished he had not come. He reminded me of all my pretensions in coming here. He was like some other sort of mirror bouncing back a reflection I didn't like—I saw myself needing this time at Bellevue to come together inside, but not daring to admit it, and pretending to be both crazy and better than I was.

"Now you can look!" Mrs. Walters turned my chair around. The hair swept down over one eye. The other side was pulled back, slick, behind the ear, only to swoop behind like a gull's wing. The top rippled with parallel rows of waves, and the mist from the hair spray settled on a creation as shiny as a brown plastic hat. Only the yellow bow, bobbing over the left ear, moved. The beauty operator framed her work with her plump hands. Earthalee and Leola, Michael and the others standing in a circle behind my chair all smiled, and I smiled, and I was beautiful.

Back on the ward Michael and I found a table in the dining room and he told me that he had spoken to the social worker and to Dr. Kegan. He had made up some story of hiring me to work in the parish office under his close supervision, and they were both pleased. Leola was hovering close by, looking for some talk with the Father, so my thanks to him were curtailed. Some perfunctory blessings, and Michael was gone.

155

During the afternoon Irene Tompkins was picked up by her husband, a stocky man with grizzled hair and an elaborate uniform. She had told me of her other husbands, and the bad marriages when she was in summer stock, or on the road. Mr. Tompkins was a different sort. She thought he was a man of substance. "We live in the temple on Delancey Street," she had told me. "He is the Grand Commander of the Save-a-Soul Mission." He looked old enough to be her father. She had convinced him to sign her out. I thought she might be on something again, for she no longer smelled of paraldehyde, and her cheerfulness was half controlled and brittle. Her husband was pompous and doting. "Isn't he wonderful?" she said on her way out. Gerta went out with her face shining. "I got a job," she said. "I'm on a weekend pass now, and next week I'm leaving for good." And at last, someone came for Jeannette Rosetti. I never said goodbye to her, for I didn't see her leave, but they told me later she was at Kings Park Hospital. There were only a dozen of us at dinner. I felt lonely and at loose ends, sorry to have missed Jeannette, but aware she wasn't thinking of me and would not miss me. Any day on the ward was filled with relationships interrupted as easily as a conversation; there were no neat endings. I knew some of these patients would be back on the ward before long, but it wouldn't be the same. I knew I and many others would be gone. I felt the irrational urge to cling to this ill-assorted group, a feeling that did not conflict with a growing excitement at the thought of leaving myself. In the meantime, there was the Sweetheart Dance to think about.

I watched Eileen Thibeau and Evelyn Howard getting ready for the dance. Their preparations took time. Eileen had something special to wear, a brightly colored jumpsuit of synthetic jersey. She borrowed Maxine's make-up and painted her cheeks red and her eyelids green and silver. When I saw how fancy she looked I got shy and wished I didn't have to go—I had a particularly baggy gown on. Only my hairdo was exactly appropriate to my situation.

An aide led us out, those of us who had off-the-ward privileges, while the other patients clustered around in envy. We might have been going to Cinderella's ball, they looked so envious. Flo Tamis was broken-hearted at being left behind until Evelyn and Phoebe promised to bring back something for her to eat, if they served refreshments.

The dance was held in a large room on the other side of the building. The ceiling was vaulted with Romanesque arches and supported by massive pillars. Letters cut from construction paper hung over the doorway: VALENTINE SWEETHEART DANCE. All around the walls were red paper hearts, some of them bearing messages like "Alphonse and Florence," or "I Love You Sweetie." One flamboyant sign said, "You the MOST!" A huge old-fashioned jukebox stood in the corner, gaudy as a carnival, flashing bright lights as the records spun. By the time we arrived the party had already begun. The guests had come from every ward except NO 2, the prison ward. It was a colorful crowd. Most of us wore hospital robes over our dresses or pajamas, but some had added personal touches. One man had tucked a bright-yellow terry-cloth towel in the neck of his pajamas as an ascot. Some of the girls wore dresses they had made in occupational therapy, or like Eileen had a dress brought from home for special occasions like this.

Some folding chairs were grouped around some of the pillars. A refreshment table held some pink punch and some sugar cookies. All the rest of the space was taken up with patients dancing. I drifted around the room picking up scraps of conversation and filing them in my mind. Patients compared conditions on men's wards and women's wards, and the women usually came off as better treated, perhaps because the female patients were more prone than the men to organize housekeeping details when the staff was short-handed, and perhaps because the female aides were generally the better trained or more satisfied with their work.

A man with a paper bag on his head staggered across the floor to me and swept me off in an elaborate gate-legged waltz. His eyes were glazed over as if he were about to fall into a fit, and I recognized him as a visitor to the ward from O 7. His legs were so much longer than mine that I couldn't keep up

157

with him, and he half lifted me every time he took a step. Before the song was over he had left me as abruptly as he found me and had taken up with someone else.

The jukebox seemed to bounce as the music got louder. Martha and the Vandellas, the Temptations, the Marvelettes. Little Richard and Bo Diddly, and Aretha Franklin's voice cutting through the din of conversation and the stomping of a hundred patients' feet like a knife wrapped in velvet.

Without warning the music ceased with an electronic shriek. The jukebox lights went out. There was a hush, and the moment might have turned to violence, the disappointment was so crushing, but several nurses and aides rushed over and rumors went out that the machine could be fixed. A couple of strong male patients were enlisted to help. After some discussion the broken jukebox was carried out like a fallen warrior and another, equally venerable, jukebox was carried in. Within fifteen minutes the music was blasting again, the jukebox was as resplendent with bright painted designs and decals and flashing blue and red lights.

In the corner Eileen was dancing with a man with golden-brown skin and eyes as green as a cat's. Otis Redding was wailing, "Will you be there, will you be there, baby? I'm lonely for you, yes I am!" Eileen and the man were moving closer, they were slithering against one another, and Eileen threw her head back and moaned. The man had her fixed with his eyes, and he ground his pelvis against hers and shook his shoulders slowly. They danced slower and more deliberately. His hands were fumbling for a way into her clothing, but the back zipper was inaccessible. The defeat didn't seem to register or, stoned on Thorazine and sex, he had lost track of time, for he tried again and again, every time the music brought his hands in range.

A man asked me to dance. He was very formal, and looked as if he expected me to reject him. His broad jaw was set defiantly, but his eyes were scared. The current dances weren't his forte, so we managed a stiff two-step. After we compared notes on our respective wards he told me his name was Robles, and he was forty-six years old. "I was in the merchant marine for fifteen years. I just got off a boat from San Francisco—that's where my mother lives, and I was excited about coming to the city. I had three nights here, and I didn't want to waste any of it, so I didn't go to sleep. I went out with some of my pals to Times Square. I can't remember very much. I had $708 in my pocket. I got into a fight and I lost it somehow. I don't remember anything until I ended up here. You'll excuse my lack of teeth." He shrugged a shoulder toward his mouth, as one hand was locked in sweaty union with mine and the other fixed to my waist. "I think I lost my plates in the fight. When I woke up here, I didn't have nothing. No dentures, no money. I didn't know who I was or why I was here. The dentures is the worst of it." His face reddened. I told him I wouldn't have noticed if he hadn't pointed out the lack, and he smiled with his lips together. I told him about my making so much noise in Washington Square, and that also seemed to comfort him.

"Funny things can happen to you and you don't know why they happen. You take me now. I don't think I was drunk, I don't think I know what the trouble was. I guess it was not getting sleep, and you see I was a little depressed. I wanted too bad to have fun. I was trying so hard because I knew I was depressed, and then is when you fuck up so bad. I beg your pardon, ma'am," he added. "Would you care for some punch?"

We wore our feelings on the sleeves of our Bellevue robes. Rarely had I been treated more like a lady. Mr. Robles offered up his manners to compensate for his lack of dentures and mental health; they were equally painful for him to acknowledge. We were so clumsy with one another, all of us, and yet we got our meaning across with far less subterfuge than in the outside world.

What a torturous joy this was, this decent human contact between the sexes. Some of the men I could see had gone weeks, months without sex, you could see it in their eyes, you could see how they avoided a direct glance, out of modesty; their need should be hidden. And so they were more polite, and

159

tense, or, finding a willing partner, tended to the corners of the room, where the dancing knit their bodies together under cover of semidarkness.

At the punch bowl I lost Mr. Robles, but found Ellis. He had Phoebe on his arm, but she was looking for Evelyn and was not pleased. Ellis taught me his special variation of the frug, and I forgot my own clumsiness; my dress was so big I moved inside with as much privacy as in a tent.

When Phoebe settled for him the next dance, I sat down beside two teen-agers from the adolescent wards. Like Masons giving each other a sign they stretched out their arms palm side up. Motionless, one's fist to the other's elbow, they stared fixedly at the two lateral lines on each wrist. On each, one of the two cuts was longer than the other, and they were as straight as if they had been drawn with a ruler instead of a razor blade. "You are healing up nicely," the boy said. He was blond and thin and perhaps seventeen years old.

"Yours is better," the girl said.

"We'll have some pretty good scars, Sally."

"Oh, my scars are in my heart," she said.

"Don't get discouraged. You've got to hang on."

Her hair was as blond as his, and as wispy, and she was very frail. "You tell me to keep my courage up, but you don't know. My Charlie has betrayed me." She spoke in a singsong that gave me the goose pimples. Her phrasing was delicate and archaic, but her inflection was picked up from street living. "I'm three months pregnant, and my Charlie has betrayed me. He went away. They won't let me out for an abortion. You tell me what you want, and I'll tell you I'm fifteen years old, and my Charlie has betrayed me."

The boy put his arms around her and rocked her back and forth. "I know, it's bad. I was so depressed that they made me live. But we'll figure something out, we'll try to. Let me help you. Just try to get better for me."

With the cruelty of her own unhappiness she ignored his affection. "But my Charlie. My Charlie is gone."

I danced with Eddie, who told me my hair was done up

pretty good, and that it was a great improvement, and with Bill. Mr. Robles found me again for the last dance. "I thought I'd lost you. I feel like it's hard to meet some of the people, not coming from these parts, being a stranger here." His honest face was so warm I swore I'd been looking all over for him. He said, "Those two look like they're having sexual intercourse," and nodded to Eileen and her partner. He blushed again. "I heard that happens sometimes. Sometimes even on the wards, they get together. It's rough, you know. The aides are pretty good at stopping that stuff, I guess. Perhaps I can come to visit you when I get out. I wish I could write down your name. My memory isn't so good since I came here." The aides unplugged the jukebox, and ward by ward we were gathered into groups and put on the elevator.

Back on the ward, Eileen was almost in a trance. "I'm in love. I told him I loved him. He's getting out, and he's going to come to see me. We've been sending notes back and forth. I wrote him a letter and told him I loved him." Evelyn said, "I saw you, little Miss Barry! You was switching your little ass around, dancing like nobody's business. You got going real good." It had been years since I had been to a dance and talked it over afterward with girls. Dances used to be bad times for a wallflower, and here unexpectedly I had been given the chance to run a dance through again, like a piece of film, but this time I felt good. I had had a nice time.

Now that it was the weekend again, Miss Rivers was back on duty. I told her about the dance, and that I was going home in the morning. "That's what happens. Everybody clears out on Friday, a few on Saturday, to make room for some more on the weekend. Already now we have a couple of ladies come in while you were at the dance; and beds fill up fast enough."

I left her to mull over the loss of the television set, and other news of the week, and stayed awake late from excitement. The next day I would be home. Jeannette's bed, at the foot of mine, was empty, and I missed her. I wondered if Priscilla was with her at Kings Park too—I had forgotten to ask. I wanted us all to be together, all of us, even Mrs. Feeny; I wanted to go home, but I didn't want to leave. I thought over what Miss Rivers said about the beds filling up, and saw the hospital fitting into life here in the city, a part of a larger system, with hundreds of patients living in the world, then filling up beds, and moving on to other beds in other hospitals, taking their turn in the world, then coming back here again, sometimes to meet again, like Evelyn and Phoebe, more often gone like Jeannette Rosetti or Sam Buck with no goodbyes said. I saw that Mrs. Briggs' bed was empty, and Gerta's. Two new patients were banging on the doors of seclusion rooms. Far from natural cycles of seed, shoot, and green leaf, we fit our own ecology. Urban detritus, every one, our lives turned in their own time. Some come, some go, and it seemed not so important after all to say goodbye.

Nine

On Saturday the sun was shining brightly outside and the snow had shrunk to dirty humps along the gutters, melting into the drains in rivers. I took my last group shower. I ate my last Bellevue breakfast. I made my bed for the last time, this time with clean fresh sheets top and bottom for some new lady.

During the morning I waited for my clothes to be sent up in their cotton bag. I talked to the new patients. One was a big, tough woman with a cauliflower ear and a nose that showed signs of having been broken in more than one place. She carried with her the smell of paraldehyde like an invisible mist. Two Band-Aids made an ex on one cheek, and her eyes were swollen almost shut. "I got in a fight in a bar on 118th Street. I got thrown out on my ass. It ain't the first time, and it'll happen again," she told me. She shook her head. "It sure was one hell of a fight. Shit, I wouldn't mind doing it all over again." Our conversation was good-humored, and it was only because I was about to go home that I imagined us meeting in the outside world. I had tended to forget during the week that among my sisters on the ward were whores and thieves, and perhaps a murderer or two as well. This woman looked as if she might have taken care of an unfaithful lover with lye.

The other new patient was tall and elegant. I would have guessed the Winsor School, and Mount Holyoke, Class of '46. Her hair was ash blond, cut simply and well just below her ears, and she ran her fingers through it over and over again. It was stringy with perspiration. "You have no idea," she said to no one at all. "You have no idea what I have been through this night. First the robbery, and now this. I've always tried to do my best, you know. I arranged affairs for charity. What more could be expected of me? I always did my best, and I had a high rate of response. The last dance netted thousands. Of course it's all gone, what with the robbery. Oh, this is a horrid, horrid place! Someone, please, direct me to the police. I've been robbed." She wore one slipper, a dirty red bootie that belonged to her, and that was encrusted with mud. The other foot was bare. The bathrobe was the one she had been admitted in, rather shabby and stained. Here one's personal habits, even one's dirty lingerie, were no secret.

Luisa's father came for her. She embraced me for the last time and told me to visit her on East Tenth and Avenue D. "I'm going back to my little baby. He is two weeks old, and I miss him so much. I will never forget you in this life," she said to me.

By noon my clothes had been sent up to me (my blue jeans were inches too big around the waist and hips, as if they belonged to someone else) and my friend Helen had come for me. There was no reason for me to be picked up, I might just as well have walked out the door by myself, and taken a bus home, but some special notice seemed fitting. Inside I could not really believe I could walk out by myself, and I was relieved I didn't have to risk it.

While Helen was talking to Miss Garber about my medication, which was a prescription of Thorazine to ease me back into daily life, Mrs. Foster pulled off her clothes in the empty dining room, and stretched out on the floor. By the time an aide reached her, the woman with the cauliflower ear was standing over her, one lazy toe slowly working around the old woman's crotch.

"Clara, now you know better than that!" Miss Jessop said. "I'm ashamed of you!"

Clara smiled, showing her broken teeth. Mrs. Foster laughed out loud. "I like that, baby!" she said. "Ooo-eee!" Miss Jessop and Miss Sendell together pulled Clara away and bundled up Mrs. Foster for seclusion. The other new patient kept talking, like a tape recorder someone had forgotten to turn off. "They used electrical beams to break in. I don't know how they did it. They were shrewd. I heard the hum of the electricity, so I know that's how they got in. They stole everything, with electrical waves."

An aide led us out the purple door and down the elevator, and through a labyrinth of tunnels and corridors, cellar hallways whose walls oozed sweat, down passages gloomy as the sewers of Paris, into the building where my property had been stored. From behind the grillwork I received an envelope. Inside were two pencils, my driver's license, my unemployment booklet, four postage stamps, and one rattail comb. It almost wasn't worth claiming. Behind me in line was a man asking for the property of a male patient. The woman behind the partition said, "But if he was D.O.A., we don't have his things. We only keep them a month here, and it's been more than a month since he was brought in. You'll have to write a letter." The man said, "He was my own brother." The woman said, "I know, but his things were sent away. You'll have to write a letter."

No one asked me about paying my bill. They were going to let me walk out. Because I was afraid this would be discovered as their mistake, and I would be apprehended at the door, I asked the woman in charge of property. She said, "Don't you worry about it now. You just get back on your feet. You'll hear sooner or later. Wait until you get a bill, and then you can work something out. There's time for that."

Outside the uneven pitches of concrete and asphalt took getting used to. I stumbled on curbs and slipped on patches of ice. Helen took me to a coffee shop nearby for my first real meal. The smells of gasoline, fresh air, food cooking, the waitress's perfume, were special and distinct. The sense of smell had been cheated more than the others this past week; my nose had nothing offered it but the odors of bodies and their functions, of linoleum corridors, of used-up cooking smells, thinned over steam tables. Like one receiving presents I touched a menu, a countertop, a plate made out of heavy china, not plastic. There was no way to communicate the feelings of getting out, nor my shyness at being out on the street. Helen was welcoming and pleased to see me and I knew I could take my time; like a diver coming up slowly to avoid the bends, I wanted to ease back into my old life. Helen's cab dropped me off at my apartment.

It didn't feel like being home. Only a week had passed, but it might have been years. The apartment was too vast for me ever to have lived in, one person in four rooms, all by herself. In the floor space here, twenty women could keep their beds in rows. And the number of belongings! The furnishings expressed a personality. Comfortable old chairs, an oriental rug in dark clear reds and blues. Enough books to last N 7 for years. N 7 had no distinctive personality, we passed in and out of beds, rooms, nightdresses, like different limbs in the same amorphous body. Having an apartment was definition, and individual. It felt peculiar not to share the riches here. There was a record player, a radio, a guitar to strum. The walls and the windows made sounds when the wind blew hard. You could see the weather out of the windows. A dog barked in the neighbor's apartment and seemed a luxury.

Nonetheless, being alone took effort. I wanted to ask permission to do the simplest things, but there was no one to ask. It was an adventure to go out of my house (remembering to lock the door behind me) and buy a paper at the newsstand on the corner. Would they let me? Would they give me that freedom? Or, conversely, would they trust me with that responsibility, to run errands all by myself? People walking to and fro on sidewalks fascinated me. I wanted to compliment them on their courage, going out alone or in small groups, and at the same time call attention to their freedom. "But you can go *anywhere you want!*"

I called some friends on the telephone, and most had not known I had been away. To one I said, "I was in Bellevue," and for response got a recital of a week's marital battles, as fully detailed as Norma June's soap-opera plots, and no reaction at all to my statement.

The afternoon was filled with errands—a trip to the A & P to cash a check, and to the laundromat. It was like my very first trip to a supermarket, my first afternoon with washing machines. How could one take these things for granted?

An old lover called by chance when I got home, to ask me to dinner, and in a French restaurant uptown I felt that this was my life after all I had walked back into, and the person who had been in the hospital and the person who had known this man were one person. Hospital routine began to slip away from me. I did not think that I was missing medication as 9:00 P.M. came and went, although from time to time in the next week, if I was tired or out of sorts, I would slip into those patterns, half waiting for someone to call me to lunch or to arrange that visitors arrive.

As the hospital experience began to recede, I feared the return of old patterns. I wondered if I, too, would soon bustle about, making too much of small matters, cutting myself off from good feelings, wasting time with dull relationships and routine. The special poignance of being free in the outside world stayed vivid for several weeks, and then it, too, began to dim.

But it was there nonetheless when I went out of my way.

167

I went up to Bellevue again, to N 7, to tell the doctors there what I had done. Falling into old habits, I had spent time worrying about Dr. Kegan's response. I thought it was important. I made up excuses for myself, and suitable rationalizations. As I was led into N 7, though, coming in through the front door, past the snack bar, up the one working elevator, all those worries fell away. I was at home here, and outside, too. On the ward some of the patients recognized me immediately. Phoebe was eager to tell me news of what had happened since I had left. There had been a knifing on the floor, an enraged husband had attacked his wife during visiting hours. The man had been apprehended as he ran outside, past guards and attendants, with no coat on, and his wife's blood on his shirt. It wasn't surprising to me. Some of the women were new, but they had problems that were familiar. Three patients came up to ask me for food, or to continue a tale they thought they had begun the day before, although we had never met until this moment. I was happy to feel no reserve here.

Dr. Kegan was not as I remembered him. Now that I was on the outside, he looked young, and pleasant enough, and not so odd as I recalled. I believed I had seen a side of him that was true, but concealed from the world in daily life; whether instead he was simply an ordinary person working at a job with some dedication seemed impossible to resolve, and unnecessary. Odds were he was both, and more, as multiple in his complexities as his patients. I knew what normal was now, if I was normal, and it implied that some life went on in him, some communication between him and patients that he might be unaware of himself, but which affected their attitudes and their recovery.

"Do you know, Miss Barry," he said, "a rumor was going around the hospital that someone was here who was observing us, and planning to write about Bellevue. We thought over who was here at that time, and we figured you were the only one it could be." I couldn't imagine how the news could have spread, for it had been a well-kept secret, but I was sure also that he was telling me the truth.

I came back several times to the ward to see patients I was close to. Once I brought some make-up from the dime store, some black eyebrow pencils, to replace those that had been stolen from Miss Pinero's cart. A couple of times I brought a bag of apples. After a while only two of my friends were still on the ward. It was much different. N.Y.U. was using Bellevue as a teaching hospital, and there were medical students on the ward and a larger staff. A huge chart was on the wall, made by some other patient, listing various levels of responsibility a patient had to achieve before he could be discharged. New partitions had gone up, making rooms where there had been none, and opening up others. There were bright posters on the walls, and many fewer seriously disturbed patients on the ward. The men and the women were mixed together during the day, all day, just as Miss Rivers had predicted. One day I paid a visit and found that Phoebe had gone home. She was the last patient from that week in February, and now it was late spring. There was no reason now for me to go back again to N 7, because it was different, it was a new place, and I had a different life. I ran into Miss Kearnes on the street, and she was not eager to talk to me. She left her crazy people in the hospital and stuck to her own business on the outside. I didn't mind at all. I knew there were no boundaries between the ward and me. Because I knew it was open, I never went back again.

Postscript

I spent one week in Bellevue, but months passed before I understood what the experience meant to me, and how it related to the reasons I went into the hospital in the first place. I had wanted to observe women in a setting that requires total dependence, and yet frees them from many of the restrictions of civility, law, and custom. Quite apart from the particular psychological or emotional aberrations that put her in Bellevue, each patient, I assumed, must respond to the very special life style of a psychiatric ward, and it was this narrow range of the "normal" reaction to such an institution that I wished to explore.

But theory, rational observation, and evaluation were inappropriate inside Bellevue. In my planning I was in the position of trying to think about being unable to think. When I went into Bellevue, I was tossing my body and my psyche down Alice's rabbit hole, and the better my reasons for doing it, the less prepared I was for the event. Any thesis at all loses meaning as soon as you enter a locked ward as a patient, for it becomes a function not of your mind, but of the expectations of the institution.

Throughout the experience I was plagued by knowing much and knowing very little, simultaneously. I knew patients would be complex, quirky, unclassifiable. Yet still I studied textbooks before I went in. I knew there would be no order or reason there that I could foresee, but this knowledge did not help my frustration when I felt cut adrift there. The more I learned on the ward, the more I had to unlearn from my past, and the less sure I became that anyone could generalize about emotional health or psychiatric institutions.

My questions when I went into Bellevue centered around the paradox of any such institution: coexisting one finds the rigid laws of locks and strait jackets and the unimaginable, lunatic freedom to choose one's own salvation. I wondered if the concepts of identity and social order would fall away on N 7, if they would be defined and enforced by the locks, or discarded by the lunatic.

We did keep our identities, and we managed to have dignity and self-respect. There was a social structure, defined partly by the staff and by certain overt and implicit rules of behavior, and even more forcefully by the patients themselves. There was a respect for idiosyncrasy hardly to be found in the outside world, along with a drift toward conformity, "getting well," and therefore being released. Certain behavior was encouraged as good, or healthy, and other behavior was bad, or sick. The staff and the patients did not always entirely agree which was which.

Few of the patients on N 7 fit neat categories. Not every patient was psychotic. Some addicts had begged or lied to get in, to kick their habit. Some senile old people might have been better cared for in a nursing home. Once, when Flo was getting on my nerves, Miss Kinney said, "Maybe she's sick, or a little slow, or both. She was in one of those halfway houses where they train you to live by yourself, but she wandered off and got into all kinds of trouble. Men in the street take advantage of her. She doesn't know they don't care about her, and she'll give them anything they want if she's not watched over. She can't take care of herself, but she's a good girl. She doesn't mean any harm. If she isn't here, where can she go? Nobody cares about girls like her, except here. What would happen to her?" Flo, with many others who have chronic or untreatable problems, shuttles between different hospitals, with short and unsuccessful forays in between to the outside world. Most hospitals end up, therefore, as a dumping ground for people who have nowhere else to go. The population is more fragmented and disorganized than any hospital's policy can deal with.

Once on the ward, the individual feels an intense pressure to justify himself for being there. One may rebel, deny one is crazy, make excuses, blame others, or, in the end, fit in and find a new kind of norm. My rationalization, that I was here not as a patient but as an observer, was not so very different from Ellis's saving face by saying he was picked up just because he was a freak. Mrs. Briggs said she was not suicidal, and therefore hauled in here by mistake. I fully believed two and three contradictory stories from each person at the same time, for I offered the same contradictions. I was indeed an observer, but being a patient was no pretense. As soon as the door was locked, I certainly *was* a patient, and the only question for me, as well as for the others, was what sort of patient I would be.

Acceptance of the foibles of other patients was one way of giving off the hope that they would respect your peculiarities as well, and it led to self-respect. One made friends with patients whose visions or delusions matched or complemented one's own. Luisa, Leola, and Jeannette held services together. Luisa, begging God to save her newborn son from some indescribable horror, would kneel with the messenger warning of Armageddon, and with the Virgin Mary, by the side of a dormitory bed, each with her palms pressed together under her chin like little children at prayers. In their tacit theological system, Leola would let Jeannette be the Virgin Mary if she in turn could be God's prophet, and bless her. In constant interaction of delusion and image, one person's vision could reinforce or alter that of another.

The patients were often self-sufficient and enterprising. If Miss Hargins wanted bread and butter in the dormitory, she put it under her dress at mealtimes. If Eileen was in love with a man on another floor, she found a way to slip a note to him. Patients took dope, disposed of medication they didn't want, got food supplies, cosmetics, cigarettes. They invented, borrowed, and stole with an efficiency that is hard to appreciate unless you know the odds against even the simplest amenities of living in a locked ward. (A year later, many improvements had bettered those odds. Now each patient keeps her possessions in a small locker on the ward, with her own combination lock. Bright yellow doors have been constructed in front of the toilet stalls, and showers are no longer communal.)

The patients' sense of individual identity overlapped with their sense of being members of a group. Although at first glance each patient did have freedom on the ward, of course there were rules enforced by the staff that limited their behavior. The staff set the routine. The times for sleeping, meals, and recreation were determined by the staff, and were arbitrary. Many of us would have liked to take catnaps during the day, and never go to bed at all. Because we had no families to care for here, and no jobs to go to, there was in fact no reason for doing our sleeping during the night. But bedtimes were early, and we were allowed to stay up late only as a special privilege, and then we were made to feel beholden. The greatest benefit of drug therapy seemed to be that some of us would sleep when sent to bed at 9:00 P.M. Without drug therapy, but with a recreation program demanding hard physical exercise, we might have been healthier and just as tranquil. (It is true that when I was on N 7 we could go into the dormitory rooms to take a nap whenever we wanted during the day. Not so very long ago dormitory doors were locked on N 7 during the day. But although the open dormitories were an innovation we appreciated, our early bedtime precluded too many naps. If we were smart, we didn't quibble with the set routine.)

Since I have left the ward, there have been many incursions on the daily routine. Patients attend more group meetings and have access to more recreational activities. Because O 7 male patients now mingle freely with the N 7 women during the day, the ward space is doubled. There is more room to move around in. One has more choice of friends and enemies. On the combined ward NO 7, a patient might have a routine different in content but not in type from daily life. He would go to bed at 9:00 P.M. after a busier day than we generally enjoyed.

The staff also determined the law. If a woman wanted to describe J. Edgar Hoover as a Communist agent calling her on his magic telephone, nobody would quarrel with her. You could say what you wanted. But if your delusion led you to smash a television set, you would pay for it by seclusion, drug therapy, or shock. When I was on the ward, guidelines to "good" behavior were implied by the staff rather than spelled out. Now the new patient's chart leaves no doubt. Before one is allowed off-the-ward privileges, one successfully copes with "1. Eating; 2. Using toilet; 3. Dressing self; 4. Not hurting self or others." The unknown patient had made explicit, by rule 8, that one must "obey hospital rules, for example a. no smoking in bed, b. no alcohol or unprescribed drugs, c. no sexual contact." The very warning against this behavior, which the staff evidently found symptomatic of "sickness," pointed up the patients' acceptance of these breaches as commonplace. The staff assumed a patient closer to help if he "participates in Activities in Daily Living Groups," and, if he co-operates, allows him to wear his own street clothes. The patient works his way up past rewards of supervised passes, snack-bar privileges, unsupervised passes, to, finally, discharge.

There was some division between the patients who agreed with the staff's standards and those who continued to hallucinate, hold delusions, deny the appropriateness of hospitalization in their case. Most patients would, like me, withdraw from the civilizing influences of ward life when they first arrived, to orient themselves and to set their defenses. They do not want to conform. If they do not pass through this stage and begin to work their way up that achievement chart on the wall, they may be sent to a state hospital for longer-term or custodial care. Miss Hargins was sent to Central Islip, and I imagine she is there still.

Some patients may never give up their unique view of themselves, but may be released anyhow. Mrs. Briggs never agreed that she was sick or that she should be in the hospital. She called her lawyer every day, including the day of her release. She did, over the course of the week, start taking her Thorazine, she stopped weeping for her dead friend, and she became less frenetic in her dealings with others. When she left the ward, her lawyer had not brought the writ of habeas corpus she had been demanding. She was released because Dr. Kegan thought she was ready to go home. His concern was less whether or not she was literally psychotic or suicidal at the time of her admission than whether or not she could now pick up her daily life again. Nonetheless, she was one of the very few who were released without in some open way "giving in" to mental health as defined by the staff. When Leola "received a sign" and began taking her medication, she also began progress toward release. Those patients who made the leap over to trusting the hospital and the staff soon might become what I thought of as "well" patients. They were exchanging their aberrations for more civilized behavior, and were eager to convince other recalcitrant patients to do likewise.

All the patients policed themselves. If Luisa was stationed at the water fountain, patients quickly helped pull her away before she caused a flood. (It was the staff, however, and perhaps a "well" patient or two, who would then lead her off to seclusion.) Patient control over each other's activities was rarely punitive. An individual act could be discouraged, such as Miss Hargins' messiness at the toilets or Priscilla's theft of cigarettes, but no patient would generalize about other characteristics from these disagreeable ones, or mock another patient for hallucinating. Women who broke rules were not made scapegoats by the other patients. Those whose habits were most offensive, and who were therefore the most difficult to spend time with, were simply left alone.

The patients constantly reinforced "good" behavior among the group. They were always teaching, supporting, counseling in small ways. The sense of shared captivity I believe was much more effective than the Thorazine in keeping the peace. It was not only my naïveté that kept me innocent of the sins of my sisters on the ward. Women who got in fights in bars would not dream of picking a fight with me. Many of the women had police records, were thieves and whores, but I was not beaten up, or assaulted sexually, and in fact no patient gave me any verbal abuse during the whole week. They were gentle and extraordinarily tactful, far less "violent," here on what used to be called the violent ward, than the equal number of women I remember from my college dormitory. (It should be noted that the old policy of isolating the disturbed patients had only recently been changed. I was put on the ward because there happened to be a bed empty there; most of the others had been hospitalized before the new system was in effect. Therefore N 7 housed a larger proportion of "violent" patients than other wards.) Distinctions of class and race and background fell away on N 7. We were not competitive. We tried not to hurt each other's feelings. The few instances of physical violence I witnessed on the ward were usually violence against property. If another patient was involved, she would be clutched or pulled at, but not hit or scratched or bitten. I had the feeling that the patients were more in control of the ward than the staff was aware of. If the patients had in one extraordinary moment chosen to rise up in rebellion, the staff would have been overwhelmed in an instant, but there was not the slightest chance that this would happen. Early enough in my stay I sensed this, and thereafter I had absolutely no fear of another patient, no matter how unorthodox her behavior.

Selena Jenks, Evelyn, or any of the other patients would describe life on N 7 very differently, and be as right as I—so I end by being tentative and without a firm opinion. Our individualism generally triumphed over our conformity, and to be fair to the variety of experience on the ward, each image should be photographed by a camera with thirty-five lenses, and thirty-five voices must overlap on a minute's length of tape. The less openly oppressive a hospital is, the better for the patients, but it is hard to know what is oppressive to all patients. I do not know if drug therapy is a very good thing. Dr. Kegan tells me that Thorazine does not merely mask psychotic symptoms; it may alleviate them. I know that medication contributed to keeping the ward calm and more cheerful than it otherwise might have been. Certainly if tractability and a quick return to one's place in society are important, drug therapy is useful. Thorazine helped and hindered my progress as a patient in ways too mysterious to chart; I know the staff was unaware of the subtleties of anxious moods, and so also unaware of how the drug affected them, what images were lost or introduced by medication.

Moreover, any medical treatment of psychosis assumes a standard for health that leaves me ambivalent. I felt that Mrs. Foster and Jeannette Rosetti, for instance, led the most vivid and meaningful lives when out of contact with conventional society. I do not know, if someone is staring into God's eye, that it is necessarily good or just to pull her back into routine life on the Lower East Side.

But here we open the locked door and let in revolution. What a ward a hospital administrator might run! If he is daring, some day it may not be a ward at all, and he may not be running it. I can imagine the ward being replaced by a commune or a collective, with staff and administrators full participants. They would share the food of those others—no longer patients—those others, who will refuse to give in. No one would be allowed to hurt another person, at any level. Politeness, except as an expression of love, would be banned. Poetry would be encouraged. To try such a radical and hopeful plan, one must first tear down the hospital, every brick. (And even now they are constructing another hospital building for the Bellevue complex, slowly enough to be obsolete when it locks up its first patients, but solid enough to last a century.)

If there are not now hands enough for the revolution, then we will settle for less. On Ward N 7, one attitude cut through ignorance, bureaucracy, and psychiatric theory. It subverted hospital policy. Because so many of us spoke in private images, we looked past words; when a nurse or an aide tried to civilize us, but showed us empathy, all her good work was undone. Love might come from a staff member or a patient, we weren't choosy. But it mattered that even here, in the purlieus of milieu therapy and resocializing behavior patterning, love sought out our devils and the magical thieves who stole from us in the night, and healed us.